TAKING AWAY THE DISTANCE

*A Young Orphan's Journey and the
AIDS Epidemic in Africa*

DISCARD

Miles Roston

CARROLL & GRAF PUBLISHERS
NEW YORK

First published in 2006 as *Kevin's Questions* by Exisle Publishing
Limited, New Zealand
First published in 2007 the United States by Carroll & Graf
Publishers, 387 Park Avenue South, New York, NY 10016.

The photograph of Kevin and Humphrey at Nyumbani and the
photograph of Jane and Kevin are both courtesy of International
Production Services, from the film *Make It Real (to me)*
Interior design by Michael Walters

A CIP catalog record for this book is available from the Library of
Congress.
ISBN-13: 978-0-7867-2082-8; ISBN-10: 0-7867-2082-4
New Zealand ISBN: 0 908988 69 9
10 9 8 7 6 5 4 3 2 1

CONTENTS

FOREWORD

Dear Friends,

To experience the stigma of being HIV positive, to care for someone you love who is living with AIDS, to bury a parent who has died from AIDS, to look into the eyes of children whose parents have succumbed to the disease—these are the realities lived and relived and relived again and again in Africa.

To many people, it is suffering they are aware of, but they are removed from it. This is a book to take away the distance. To raise awareness of the awful realities of this disease and its consequences. We are made for togetherness, members of one family in God's global village. We are all affected by this disease, and its consequences will haunt all our futures.

I commend Miles Roston for the outstanding work he is doing to encourage us to reach out to our sisters and brothers with compassion, and of course the young and courageous Kevin Sumba. Together, they are asking the difficult questions of each of us: what will we all do to help the millions of children affected by this epidemic, and what will we do to prevent more millions of children from being orphaned?

God bless you

-Desmond M Tutu, Archbishop Emeritus
June 2006

Does it matter to anyone if there is one less of us?

Does it matter if any of us live or die?

PROLOGUE

HAPPY BEGINNINGS

Orphan c. 1300, from L.L. orphanus "parentless child" (cf. O. Fr. Orfeno, It. Orfano), from Gk. Orphanos "orphaned," lit. "deprived," from orphos "bereft" . . .

This is a book about HIV/AIDS that actually has some happy endings. For millions of people—adults and children—suffering the effects and the fallout of this dreaded disease, there is far too much misery, with no happy endings to their stories these days. But there can be. There can be many more happy endings, and beginnings.

I have traveled across our globe to meet people who have been affected by this disease, from leaders and scientists to local workers and patients, including a man who died the day after I last saw him because he did not have medicine. That was how I started to become affected. To quote a heroic nurse in a ward of dying patients, "Even if you are not infected, we are affected so much."

Most of all, I became affected by the children I've met who were affected so much by this disease, children left to live alone because of their parents' deaths, some HIV positive themselves. There are over fifteen million of these children worldwide, the majority of them in sub-Saharan Africa. By 2010, some estimates say there will be eighteen million. And there are forty million-plus people living with HIV/AIDS worldwide; twenty-five million people have died of the disease at the time of writing—twenty-five million individual human beings.

Numbers can mean so little these days. Statistics are hard to relate to. But here are some ways to think about it. The population of California is about thirty-six and a half million. One whole California is not equal to all the HIV positive people in the world. Texas has a population of twenty-three and a half million. One Texas is not even equivalent to all those who have died.

In terms of AIDS orphans, think of New York state, with a population of nineteen million. Poof! Imagine it in 2010 magically as an AIDS orphan country—literally only filled with children whose parents have died because of this torturous disease.

France and the United Kingdom have a population of sixty million each. Imagine one-third of these as orphaned children. Imagine in 2010 half of the population dead.

Even imagining HIV/AIDS and its effect on children this way doesn't really bring home the enormity of this disease's impact. It still doesn't encapsulate the suffering of these millions of individual human beings—the loneliness the children endure, or the amount of discrimination and fear they encounter in their communities.

Though I traveled among these children, I didn't really feel this disease myself until I allowed myself to be affected so much by one child. A boy named Kevin.

CHAPTER ONE

MEETING KEVIN SUMBA

I had a brief. I was finally to do a film on HIV/AIDS for a group of nonprofit organizations, which in turn were funded by the Bill and Melinda Gates Foundation. My fiancée, Sarah Lambert, also a filmmaker, and I were partners in a small New York-based production company. We had been trying to get films about the epidemic funded for years, notably a film about the race for an AIDS vaccine, but to no avail.

On some level, our attachment to the cause was personal. Sarah had grown up as a child actress in Australia, where many of her friends and members of the theater and film community were stricken with the disease. I'd grown up in New York with my parents and younger brother and sister. Though my father and mother were often poor in money, they got us—via scholarships—into an alternative private Waldorf school. I'd come of age in the '80s, when the HIV/AIDS epidemic was raging through the arts community. (And I'd had the privilege of developing projects with John Glines, who produced the well-known play about AIDS, *As Is*.) Now I was a supposed grown-up in this production company focusing on social issues for adults and children alike. But raising any money for a film on the realities of HIV/AIDS seemed nigh on impossible. (Ironic, really, in the age of reality television.)

However, in 2001, through the World Conference on Religion and Peace—an organization working with the commonalities of all religions, and whom we'd done films for previously—partnering with four other organizations to help orphaned and vulnerable children, we would at last get to make a film on the epidemic, focusing on the AIDS orphans. I would direct it, due to my experience in Sierra Leone in West Africa. (At the time, Sarah and I were also working with children worldwide, directing an animated and live-action sixty-five-part series called *Aliens Among Us*, which starred real children and an alien, a little less real.) Sarah would produce from our offices in New York.

For this first shoot, I was working with the NGO consortium's media representative, Beatrice, from Italy, as well as a local crew and Christian, a cameraman from New York. We were looking for children orphaned by the epidemic, to film their stories and show the problems created by the disease, especially in the poorer areas struck by HIV/AIDS. The idea was that somehow, by showing the stories of the children affected by AIDS, we could cut through the extraordinary swath of conflicting feelings and taboos surrounding the epidemic.

After all, this disease is special, to put it mildly. It is mainly transmitted when human beings have sexual intercourse. With thousands of years of religious and cultural prohibitions regarding sex, we as human beings have been unable to rise to the pandemic's challenge: to approach people who have acquired this disease through sex without the weight of those thousands of years of judgments and prejudices. In some sense, we still blame the victim in regard to AIDS.

But children are innocent, right?

Children whose parents have died or have HIV can't be blamed by any of us, can they? In this film, we hoped that perhaps by looking at the "innocent" victims of the epidemic, we humans—including myself—could find a way toward finding compassion without condemnation toward anyone caught in the midst of this epidemic.

Along with a local crew, Beatrice, Christian, and I went to Kisumu, the biggest town in Western Kenya, right on Lake Victoria. This area had been hit especially hard by the epidemic. There, we went into a slum called Pandipieri and visited the Pandipieri Catholic Centre, a compound of a few simple buildings set in the midst of the clutter of clay shacks that formed the community. This was a local organization founded by a Dutch priest named Father Hans that had been highlighted by people in the capital of the country, Nairobi, as actually doing something concrete in its community. (Pandipieri, I was told, literally meant "watch your backside.")

In a tiny room upstairs in this slum, we explained what we were looking for to Nathalie, a strawberry-blonde young woman in her thirties from the Netherlands, then in charge of the center. Also with us was Sister Bernadette, an Irish woman in her late fifties, and Joseph, a slender young local Kenyan man who looked maybe twenty-two or twenty-three. I was surprised to hear that, as young as he was, he was the Pandipieri counselor.

We told them we were hoping to meet and get to know and film children orphaned by the HIV/AIDS epidemic. I explained that I'd been working with children on a children's series, turning their own stories into dramas starring themselves, with the process itself being fun. With this particular project, we wanted to create an experience that could be similarly fun for the child, but at the same time moving for adult viewers.

Christian, Beatrice, and I listened as Nathalie, Joseph, and Sister Bernadette discussed the possibilities. They nodded most when discussing one boy whom they had recently come across. He was a twelve-year-old whose mother had died of AIDS and who now, unlike the majority of such children, lived alone. Joseph had just begun counseling him, and had learned of him through a teacher at a local elementary school. His name was Kevin.

We drove down the main road a bit, past people bicycling and goats meandering, then walked through a series of clay shacks with tin roofs, surrounded by piles of muck and stray garbage, in which large pigs and scrawny chickens rooted around. We passed food stalls of old timber, where tomatoes, onions, and other vegetables were being sold. In a tiny enclosure, a man—the local "butcher"—roasted meat over the ground.

The competing sounds of African reggae and religious hymns blared from various shacks.

One drunk old man latched on to Beatrice, who kept on trying to explain to him what it was we were trying to do. In reality, he could not understand. Here were a bunch of *muzungus* (white people) with some modestly well-off Kenyans and two video cameras wandering around his neighborhood. What were we doing there, in an area where even the police didn't often go?

Kids peered out from underneath their mothers' skirts, women washing the laundry in blue plastic buckets. They seemed so curious about us, which I thought odd. As this place was the epicenter of the epidemic in Kenya, surely they were used to journalists crawling over it? Surely they were used to cameras? No, that wasn't the case.

As we walked, Joseph told me about his own life; he had been selling secondhand clothes on the street before getting a job with Pandipieri and finally being promoted to counselor with only a modicum of training. At least, he said, he lived in the same community (he pointed over the shacks toward his home), so he understood what they were going through.

Hidden away in a small courtyard was Kevin's little shack made of cracked brown clay walls, a rusting corrugated tin roof, and a green door. Neighbors watched us as we approached: small children dressed only in T-shirts, an older woman scrubbing clothes in a washbasin, and another woman a few shacks down just lying on a mattress on the ground.

Kevin came to the door. He was dressed in a frayed but impeccably clean white shirt and khaki shorts—his school uniform. This thin twelve-year-old boy was ever in that school uniform. After Joseph explained who we were, we entered Kevin's home and sat with him. He had a small front room with wooden slats for windows (which looked out onto the back of the alley—basically, the latrine). The walls were of mud, but the place was clean and tidy. He had a coffee table, surrounded, oddly enough, by seven chairs. A lot of chairs for one boy living by himself. (I found out later that they belonged to his mother. When I asked him why he didn't sell them, he just looked at me as if I were crazy. He couldn't sell them: "They belonged to my mother.") In the back was a small dark room with just enough room for his bed and a tiny lamp.

Joseph told Kevin who we were, and prodded Kevin to tell us some of his story. The boy began very reluctantly, in monosyllables for the most part, answering our questions translated through Joseph into Swahili. He seemed a child wounded beyond measure, but who could not or would not expose it; indeed, the wound was almost too dangerous to expose. Throughout the week that we spent with him on this first trip, he would remain shy, unable to open up, but we managed to piece together some of the basic elements of his story.

Kevin's mother had died about two years previously. I don't remember him saying of what then, although we knew that it was of HIV/AIDS. That was of course something he could not disclose to the community at large.

There was a simple funeral. Afterward, an aunt (although I was later to learn that, in this culture, an older woman who is a friend of the family is often called an aunt) had remained with

Kevin to take care of him. However, after a few weeks, Kevin came home from school one day to find her gone. None of the neighbors knew where she went.

From that day on, he lived on his own.

To make money, he would go to the open-air markets and buy raw peanuts for some thirty-odd shillings. In his shack, he would then roast the peanuts in a pan, salting them, and cooking them over a paraffin stove. He would bring them to a woman who had been a friend of his mother. The woman sold the peanuts along with her other wares by the lake, where the fishermen gathered in the mornings with their small blue boats and hand-drawn nets. Then, a few times a week, he would pick up the money from her back in town, where she sold second-hand clothes later in the day. He would get about 150 shillings. (At the time, the exchange rate was about seventy-eight shillings to the U.S. dollar.)

At this time, primary school in Kenya cost far more than someone like Kevin could obviously afford. Besides books, there were also tuition and other sundry fees. Having the uniform, and desperate to stay in school, he snuck into the classroom every day, avoiding any time when roll calls would be taken or fees requested.

At night, he would come back home to his shack and cook himself sukamaweeki when there was money for food. (Sukamaweeki, literally meaning "pushing the week," is basically chopped kale, which if you "push" it can last you the week.) Kevin would sit at his little coffee table surrounded by his mother's chairs. He would study if he had money for paraffin and then go to sleep every night, as he did acknowledge, "very lonely."

This was how Kevin had survived, roasting these peanuts about twice a week for the last two years, with no counselor to talk to. None of the teachers in school knew that he was living alone or that his mother had died. He had presumably attended church, because he seemed religious, but didn't seem to be connected to any of the priests there.

He told us all this over a period of days. One night at his shack as he spoke to us, a neighborhood chicken came in, clucking. At times the chicken was louder than poor shy Kevin. As night drew near, the chicken insisted on coming in and out, in and out, as we left the door open for the last light we could get for filming.

I remember Kevin well at this moment, lit only by the paraffin lamp—a little boy alone in a shack. Alone.

The reason his plight had been discovered was that one day his teacher, Miss Nancy Otieno, had asked him to come along to help clean a church with some classmates. He had told her that he couldn't, as he had to go and see a woman in town. When she asked why, he told her he had to pick up money. When she began pressing as to why he had to pick up money, she had seen the tears start from his eyes. That's when he'd told her his story. This had happened only a few weeks prior to our meeting him.

Kevin's teacher had called Pandipieri Catholic Centre, and that's when Joseph had been brought in, so Kevin would at least have someone to speak to, to confide in. The teachers and the headmaster at school were looking for a way to get Kevin's school fees paid, even considering whether they might collect contributions from the parents of other kids at the school who could afford it. This was something they'd done for other orphans, but it was getting difficult now, as there were ever-increasing numbers of these children.

With the local Kenyan crew (Wanjuhi and Stephen), we filmed Kevin's story. We re-created his life: going to the market and buying peanuts, roasting them, living by himself, walking to school by himself. Early on, Stephen acted as "translator." Those who know me well know that at the best of times I am a complete mumbler. When I first started directing Kevin, it went like this. I would say, "Kevin, can you move your chair and then go to the stove?" But instead of translating my English into Swahili, Stephen would just repeat in English what I had said—only with a Kenyan accent! That, Kevin seemed to understand.

We had a good time filming. Kevin even laughed sometimes in his shy, lost way. And it seemed that as a result of our filming, he would now definitely be able to stay in school.

But this was not one of the happy endings I mentioned earlier. This was not an ending at all. This was just a beginning.

I didn't know at this point that this boy, who it seemed did not speak "Milesian" English, would play such an important part in my own life in the years to come.

CHAPTER TWO
ORPHANS ON OPRAH

When I returned to New York and looked at the footage of the various filming we had done with Kevin and other children in Kisumu, Mombasa, and Malawi, I found their stories as incredibly moving as I'd felt them to be when filming. However, other people I showed them to, most importantly my producer (and remember, fiancée), Sarah, couldn't see what I had. She saw that I had seen and felt their suffering, and she felt it, too. But she pointed out, on film, they looked like they were fine. As a child actress herself, she understood that, how a child could look fine, whether they were or not.

Even Valentine, a twelve-year-old girl at Kevin's school, looked "fine." She had lost her mother two years earlier, her stepmother a year ago, and her father only two weeks before we had met and filmed her.

Even a five-year-old boy named Stephen, whose mother had died and whose father, now sick, was drinking heavily, looked "fine." Stephen had to take care of his three-year-old HIV-positive brother, Philomon. They were fed beans by Joseph at Pandipieri, and smiled as they ate. On camera, they all seemed "fine."

My editor, the ever-agreeable Anna Laffy, also an Australian but from Melbourne, agreed with Sarah.

And though I railed at Sarah at the office and at home, I had to admit (privately!) that she was right.

This was an important lesson for me in terms of understanding children orphaned by the epidemic. The orphans I met had learned to do what we adults do when asked how we are. We say we're "fine"—no matter how we're feeling. We act like we're fine. (As the song goes, "Smile, though your heart is breaking . . .")

We're adults. We know how to lie.

These children had become little adults. Kevin and Valentine at twelve. Stephen at five. Because there were no adults to shield them, they became the adults themselves. They mimicked us. They lied.

I had seen their situation; I had been horrified. I had seen how frail Kevin was, how small Stephen was, how vulnerable Valentine was, but it did not come across on film. They did not cry needily on cue as television-savvy Americans have learned to do. The children appeared self-sufficient, far older than their actual ages; people assumed Stephen was not five but ten. This was especially true of the street kids we filmed. They acted with so much bravado.

Though our audience might intellectually understand that it would be difficult for such young children to go through life on their own, we didn't have a film that would show that emotion. I had not delved that far into the children's lives. Why not? To protect them? Or to protect myself from getting too affected? Or attached?

The NGO clients and Beatrice were happy with the short message film we had cut for them, a film to be shown to a conference in Nairobi of religious leaders from across Africa and then distributed and used for fund-raising. But we did not have anywhere near what we needed for a film broadcast to millions of people. I needed footage that would show these kids' emotions or else the message that they were actually in trouble would not come across.

Luckily, we had already planned to film the religious leaders' conference and would not be far from Kevin and Kisumu, and the other children in Kenya.

Most importantly, Sarah gave me firm instructions that when I returned there, at all times I must keep her voice in my ear: her voice telling me to get the children's emotional lives on camera, even if it made them or me cry. In order for us to make a real difference in their lives, the reality of their lives, their emotional lives, needed to come across—on-screen. I had to do much more than merely scratch the surface with them. I had to affect them; which meant I had to be affected.

Christian later asked me what had changed my way of interviewing them. I replied, "Sarah's voice in my ear!"

That ended up changing not only my way of interviewing, but also me.

CHAPTER THREE
RETURN TO KEVIN

So I returned to Kisumu two months later, with Christian. It would be just the two of us on this trip. I knew that we would be able to get to know the children better with a smaller crew. That perhaps this way, the children could be more open about their feelings on the hardships they'd gone through. When we got there, I explained this to Joseph, the counselor. He in turn explained, as he had the last time, that it was not his people's way to discuss bad things—an approach that I found odd in a counselor. I told him that, in my experience, based on my past interviews with child soldiers in Sierra Leone, it would actually help these kids to talk about their trauma.

When we arrived at his shack, Kevin seemed pleased to see us, and very surprised. I asked him why. He replied by asking where Valentine was. I asked him why. Then he admitted he had thought that we had taken Valentine with us. He seemed almost envious for a moment. I told him we didn't know where she was. Then that look disappeared, as Valentine had not long after our first visit. (When we checked to see what had happened, her teacher told us that she, maybe now all of thirteen, had got into trouble with boys, sleeping with them, and had left. The school had no idea how to get in touch with her. However, we, on that trip at least, found her living in the country with her rural family.)

As I was now more up to the challenge, willing to prod, willing to ask how it felt, and had actually returned, Kevin told me more. He wasn't a willing American *Oprah* guest, but, as a result of spending more time together, he did begin to tell me more than how to roast peanuts. And I learned that he could speak English well, and even understand Milesian!

With minor translation.

He told me mostly how lonely he was. How he couldn't stand to look at the few photos of his mother that he had, as that made him remember. It made him remember how she used to tell him and his sister stories before they went to bed at night. He was referring to his younger sister, who had been taken in by his uncle after his mother's funeral. His sole uncle lived in Eldoret, five hours away by bus. His older brother lived up there, too. They had all left Kevin on his own.

I couldn't understand how they could have just left him. I couldn't imagine my brother and sister doing that to me. In terms of relatives, I didn't really have anything to compare his situation to except my large extended family, which might have been lost fifty years earlier during the Holocaust. At the time,

Kevin couldn't or wouldn't explain it, either. Much later, I found out that the uncle had lost his job and now worked selling odds and ends, barely able to make ends meet for his family. So perhaps he had felt he could only take care of the sister. Kevin's older brother had had to drop out of school. (In a way, maybe he envied Kevin: he at least was still going to school, even if he had just been sneaking in.)

Kevin talked about his life in a language all his own. "The day I'm not going to eat sometimes I don't have something to use—like money. Or there is nothing to be cooked. So when they're there, I can prepare them and eat. But when they're not there, I can just stay like that and wait for the next day. If it will be found, it will be eaten."

He explained how difficult it was when he got sick. Over and over, he talked to me about how lonely he was. "Very lonely," he said.

I asked Kevin what he wanted to be when he grew up. He wanted to be a doctor. An AIDS doctor.

One of the conceits in this film was to give each child the opportunity to be what they dreamed of becoming. In this way, we adults would see what these children could be if they were given the opportunity to achieve their dreams. This was why we called the film *14 Million Dreams,* for the fourteen million HIV/AIDS orphans at the time.

On our earlier trip, Wanjuhi had gained access to a local hospital and clinic. We put Kevin into a white lab coat, with a stethoscope. For one afternoon, he got to be a twelve-year-old doctor. We loaned him a mobile phone to use as if he were on call as he walked in the hallway. Then, in the doctor's office, he took Wanjuhi's blood pressure. Afterward, sitting behind his desk, he wrote her a prescription and handed it to her. In the background, we could hear kids crying, patients shuffling, nurses calling—a real clinic.

Kevin had smiled a lot that afternoon. A lot.

(In the film, Valentine got to be a teacher. The boy named Jimmy in Malawi learned to drive. Ann Njeri from Mombasa got to be a nurse and her friend Evelyn Shiro a jet pilot—in a 727 plane donated for the morning by a very kind man, Ken Ahkoko, at Air Kenya! Donated literally with only a day's notice and giving us use of the whole airport!)

Of all of these children, though, I felt for Kevin most. Ann and Evelyn had Lucy Yinda, an extraordinary woman who had founded and ran Wema Centre, a home for street children. Jimmy had a rural village to look after him, and foster parents. Valentine even had a grandfather who wanted her to finish school. All Kevin had was what was loosely called his "community." Yet he still lived on his own.

When it came time to say goodbye to Kevin, I remember feeling a deep sadness. As we drove him through the night to Pandipieri, Kevin and I promised to write to each other. When we dropped Kevin off near his shack, he and I hugged, as stalls sold kale, tomatoes, and onions by paraffin lamps. Then he disappeared into their midst.

Leaving Kisumu and Kevin for what I thought then was for good, I spoke with Joseph, the counselor, and others in the community about what could best be done for Kevin and for the other children we had filmed. We wanted to make sure they would all have good lives. But we wanted, and it seemed imperative, to do things according to what the Kenyans, the community, would feel was right.

Over and over, as we had been making this film and talking about the problem of the orphans, everyone would comment that you can't build orphanages for fourteen million children. These are not Dickensian times, people would say. The children should stay within the community, within their cultural heritage and in their communities. So it was decided that when Kevin finished primary school, he should still continue to live in Kisumu. In his shack. In his community. And then have his secondary school paid for. That that's what he would wish for. It was also what he said he wished for at the time. Everyone agreed that this would be best for him. It was the accepted wisdom.

I found out years later that we were wrong.

I was wrong.

Kevin, I apologize.

CHAPTER FOUR

UNABLE TO RETURN

I returned to New York City. Within months, I finished the film. Finished the job. With the consortium of NGOs, Beatrice made sure that Kevin's school fees were taken care of. Kevin and I corresponded by letter from time to time.

Besides making its debut on television on the Sundance Channel, through the efforts of a supporter and new friend, Keri Douglas, the film premiered at the National Press Club in December 2003, at the Senate building. Keri, who later began working with an AIDS organization herself, also organized a wonderful big AIDS charity event in Washington, D.C., and in Chicago. It was called "Sweet Charity." Dessert chefs donated their time and extraordinary recipes for an evening event devoted to the children. (Sweets and children seemed a natural match.) As a speaker, I got to harangue invited senators, congressmen, and people in the administration. Somewhat like a child myself, I naïvely believed somehow that the film *14 Million Dreams* would make a real difference. Or that my tirades would.

But the disease didn't go away. The orphans did not go away.

My sister Carmel had told me how her son, then some three years old, who normally liked the water, one day became scared of going to swim in the ocean. To reassure him, she said it would "hold him." He threw a fit, screaming that it would not hold him. Finally, she tenderly asked why. He told her the ocean couldn't hold him. It didn't have arms. Not like hers.

Our world had left these millions of orphans to swim in an ocean with no arms to hold them.

I tried to return to normal, whatever that is. I didn't know anymore.

In the meantime, our production company broke up, unpleasantly to say the least. Recriminations unfortunately flew between our then business partner on the one hand and Sarah and I on the other. It was painful. I've since been told that company breakups can be worse than divorces.

Sarah and I did one more film in the United States, codirecting a film about the religious right's influence on the administration of George W. Bush. We included a section about AIDS and Africa, of course. We decided to move to other countries: to her native Australia, to Amsterdam, and to Australia again. We would start again. Afresh. I would work on (what I think is) a lovely fantasy film I'd been dreaming about for years. I would write. Swim. Cook.

I had done my bit for the AIDS epidemic. That was it. I

didn't want these children and their fourteen million dreams taking up my dreams anymore, endlessly calling in my sleep. But they wouldn't stop calling. Especially one lonely boy, who in my mind stayed twelve years old, alone, lonely, reading by a paraffin lamp in a shack far away.

I could have found other subjects to work on. I had many in mind—for children's projects, for adult dramas, for documentaries. But I dropped them.

Why?

I couldn't understand—childishly, ironically perhaps—why people weren't furious about the fact that millions of children were growing up this way, alone, many helpless. Terrorists in the Middle East and elsewhere could make headlines on a daily basis, but this epidemic was perceived as boring.

Yet all these years into the HIV/AIDS epidemic, there seemed to be no improvement in the lives of all these millions of children, an estimated fourteen million at that point. In the United States, President George W. Bush had talked about a big commitment of funds to HIV/AIDS medicines and to prevention, but as of spring 2004 these billions of dollars had yet to be released.

In governments and in organizations around the world, there was a lot of talk about a new acronym: OVCs (Orphans and Vulnerable Children). There were conferences. There were meetings. But there were many more children like Kevin.

I had to make another film about the children. I had to get to know Kevin better. What his struggle was. I had to fathom whether the universe, like the ocean, did or did not have arms to carry these children when they fell. Because, so many times, when things went badly for me, it had seemed that it didn't. And I had the support of my parents, my siblings, Sarah. What then must it be like for Kevin, alone in that universe?

Perhaps I can put it more simply. I needed to know if our lives mattered. And mine had seemed to matter just a little bit more when I helped to slightly aid the fate of one small twelve-year-old in Kisumu, Kenya, thousands of miles from the place I was born.

To make another film about these children didn't actually feel like a choice. It felt like until I made it I would be choking. Breathing would only be possible with it. Even if I could swim.

CHAPTER FIVE

KEVIN'S NEXT JOURNEY BEGINS

Nathalie and her husband, Frederik, who had worked with the Pandipieri street children rescue program, had left the Catholic Centre to work on the epidemic with other organizations. Frederik also founded his own organization, Share People. But they stayed in their adopted home of Kisumu, in close contact with Pandipieri, and in touch with Kevin via Joseph. Through Nathalie and Frederik, I began to e-mail Kevin.

At Keri Douglas's charity benefits, a pamphlet had been distributed. In it there was a quote from my friend Pierre Peyrot, a filmmaker and journalist long devoted to fighting the AIDS epidemic and a quote from me. I had also asked Kevin, through Nathalie, if he had a thought he wanted to share with these congressmen, senators, and others. His response had been typed up by Frederik, so that all the way from Kenya, Kevin, now fourteen years old, could communicate directly with decision-makers.

He had written:

*What being an AIDS orphan is—my experience: Being
an orphan is one of the unforgettable things in a human
life, as it involves losing both loved ones. As an orphan
you never know what the day might bring. I might go
hungry at times because someone can't provide for me. I
fear dropping out of school, because I can't pay the fee,
and people taking advantage and forcing me into labor.*

He was still scared, still afraid of the universe. And how
indeed could the universe protect him? Where he lived, 40 percent of women in his age-group were HIV positive.

As Sarah and I prepared to leave the United States, Pierre
Peyrot and I talked about how we could make a different film,
with more impact, to see just what people were doing about the
epidemic. Pierre had been one of the executive producers of
Steps for the Future, thirty-nine films made by sub-Saharan
African filmmakers about the AIDS epidemic. He had also
been the media manager at the last four International AIDS
Conferences.

In *14 Million Dreams,* Kevin had moved not only me but also
quite a few viewers as well. We had made a small difference,
giving people a look into the world that children like him
inhabited. But in that film, he had appeared as he was then: a
victim, a boy impacted and now surviving—heroically.

What if we could give Kevin a voice, a film in which he could
really confront the leaders of his time, all the way from the
slums of Kisumu? What if, instead of us interviewing him, he

could interview us? It was one thing for me, a supposedly grown-up adult, to ask the questions. It was quite another for a child orphaned by AIDS to do the asking. What if people, just like in the pamphlet, could be confronted by Kevin, by one of fourteen million children who had no voice with which to confront the leaders of the world? What if Kevin could lead an investigation to discover how he could protect himself from the epidemic and what people worldwide indeed were doing about it?

Via e-mail, I asked Kevin if he was interested. I told him we were determined to go to the International AIDS Conference no matter what. Would he be interested in writing questions for world leaders that we could ask there? (I had no idea how we would afford to go, but just in case . . .)

Kevin said yes; he was very much interested, and he wrote the following questions for me to ask. Frederik scanned them and then e-mailed them to me in Australia.

In his way, Kevin called his questions "Answers."

Kevin's Answers:

Questions I have and if I could ask world leaders and government officials and members of the US congress about AIDS is that:

What will they do when they realize that in a certain region three-quarters of people have been affected by AIDS? What will they do to save the lives of the remaining quarter?

What will they do to ensure that statistics of AIDS do not rise further in such a region?

How and what responsibilities will they take to ensure those affected live longer and lead a normal life full of happiness and not sorrow and suffering?

What responsibility will they take to ensure that those left do not suffer much, especially orphans?

How can they create AIDS awareness to areas where people are illiterate and believe that AIDS does not exist but is caused by breaking of taboos?

Most people with AIDS are always neglected and feared because people believe that if you associate with them you can be affected.

Orphans left behind suffer more because nobody cares for them and those taken by relatives as guardians are mistreated as some are forced into early marriages especially girls, while boys are sent to work or to be street children.

I am curious to know about other teenagers of my age in other countries because we share a lot in common in that we orphans do not have parental love, we are lonely and distressed most of the time. I suppose teenagers in England, France and America also go through similar experience, and I care very much as we are one.

Life in other places I suppose is better than the one I am leading. And I am very eager to know about it so that I can compare.

Being in school is important for me in that it gives me an opportunity to get focused and work to achieve my goals which will enable me to be of service in the future. It is also where I have a lot of friends whom I interact with and share our problems [and] dreams, [and] discuss and solve them. School is where I am always happy, because as I interact with others it makes me forget the past, which makes me feel lonely most of the time.

What I would like to be done for me to make life better is that I be provided with all basic needs, which I lack most, and especially education and learning materials. Like textbooks.

Idea I had on how to make the world a better place especially for those who suffer, departed and the needy is to help them overcome their suffering by providing them with basic needs they lack.

What I feel in my heart now is that I am relieved of some suffering and I am happy about it and hope it will be much better.

At this point, no broadcaster or organization had put up any funds or committed to our project. But Pierre and I didn't want to lose the opportunity of filming at the International AIDS Conference, where people devoted to fighting the epidemic would gather from around the world. Pierre would be there anyway in the capacity of media manager and could arrange press access. The event was crucial to making our film. If we didn't shoot at this conference, we would have to wait two more years for the next one. And now we had in our hands . . . Kevin's questions!

So Pierre and I determined we would pay the costs of the trip out of funds from what we called the Pierre Peyrot Foundation and the Miles Roston Foundation—i.e., our tapped-out bank accounts and credit cards. Keri Douglas charitably donated $1,000 toward the costs as well. Given that Sarah and Pierre's wife, Lieke, had to work harder to supplement our incomes, they suggested that a title card in the film should read that funding was from the Sarah Lambert and Lieke Krijnen Foundation.

A Finnish cameraman, a friend of Pierre's, would help us

film. We would have filmed on Scotch tape if necessary (and ended up shooting some demonstrations with the video portion of my little digital camera).

In July 2004, I boarded a plane for Bangkok.

The theme of the International AIDS Conference was "Access For All." More than seventeen thousand people gathered in Bangkok, including luminaries such as Mary Robinson (former president of Ireland and UN Commissioner of Human Rights); Thoraya Obaid, head of the United Nations Population Fund (UNFPA); and even Nelson Mandela; as well as scientists, representatives, and heads of huge pharmaceutical companies such as Roche and Glaxo Smith Klein; activists protesting those pharmaceutical companies; people victimized by the epidemic living with HIV/AIDS; nurses from Ohio; and a financier with an orphanage in China for a town where there were no parents left at all. (Ironically, it turned out he and I had both gone to college at Columbia University and actually graduated the same year.)

The conference was hosted by Senator Mechai Viravaidya, who'd been nicknamed "Mr. Condom" in Thailand for years, due to his endless fight against the AIDS epidemic through promoting condoms. He'd even started a restaurant called Condoms and Cabbages. His daughter, Sujima, was head of the youth component of the conference. And there were many youth activists, all wondering why an adult generation would not listen to them, considering they were the ones most impacted by this disease.

In the madness of the conference, with Thai dancers on stages in the entrances, with thousands of people walking to and fro, with huge pharmaceutical stands contrasted with demonstrations against those same pharmaceutical companies, patent policies, and/or the United States government, I asked people Kevin's questions. This, after all, was the point: here were people from everywhere and all walks of life dedicated to fighting the epidemic that had irrevocably changed him and millions like him.

I spoke to an elderly female doctor from India who upheld the prominent abstinence message for young people, which was being promoted by the Bush administration, among others. She said she'd been fighting the epidemic for over ten years.

I also met a sex worker from India. Middle-aged, dressed in a blue sari, she was at a stand of sex workers united in wanting to stop the AIDS epidemic, from Brazil, from Cambodia, wherever they could organize. She was angry with the American president and the ABC (Abstain, Be faithful, Condomize) argument. "Sex work exists as a profession; it always has existed. And one of the reasons is that men come to the women to buy sex."

She insisted she always used condoms now. "I refuse customers who want to have sex without condoms."

To religious and political leaders around the world who were saying "abstain abstain abstain," she responded, "ABC is absolutely wrong. It can never work. This will actually harm sex workers doubly. They will become more vulnerable to infection. And they will become more destitute and poorer. They will be forced to go off the streets, go underground, or not work. And what will happen to our children, our parents, and our families whom we support through sex work?"

I spoke with a representative of the American administration, who was angry that so many people were demonstrating against Bush's plan in which the United States would aid fifteen countries of its choosing. He said he was ready to pack up and go home. He certainly didn't want to be interviewed on camera.

I spoke to a student who was one of those demonstrating against the president's plan. He complained that the money was mainly going to campaigns stressing abstinence, and felt that instead of picking and choosing which country to help, the U.S. government should offer assistance unilaterally.

I spoke to a young homosexual Thai man who was HIV positive, who said he had been discriminated against when looking for work. So he had founded an organization for young infected Thais.

I spoke to a nurse from Ohio, part of an American group of nurses treating HIV patients.

To an ACT-UP activist from Paris.

To Kenyan social workers.

To Zimbabweans, South Africans, Cambodians, Australians.

I met Christopher Murray, a strong stout man in his fifties from Roche Pharmaceuticals, and posed Kevin's questions to him. He was director of the International Division, overseeing all Roche's activities in the Middle East, the Indian subcontinent, and Africa. "Our role is to develop and to produce and to make products available," he said, saying they had reduced their prices to cost in the developing countries, very aware of the accusations against pharmaceutical companies trying to profit from the disease (in our modern societies that insist on profits).

"But if there's not enough funding available, this is obviously a problem. And that is where I think we are today in Africa. There is not sufficient funding available for the health-care systems to take up the medication from the manufacturers, be it from generic manufacturers or research-based companies."

I commented, "The problem is that AIDS is very slow. It's years in the making. So it doesn't look as exciting as a war. But is it an emergency?"

"It's worse than an emergency," he said. "We passed the emergency phase. I mean, we should have been doing different things a long time ago. But we haven't. And the message to get across to everybody is, stay HIV negative. I mean, prevention is better than cure. There's no question about that."

His colleague David Reddy, head of research for Roche, confirmed that there was no cure at the moment, in case there was any doubt.

In front of a poster proposing lemon juice as a possible preventative tool in a room of literally thousands of scientific posters, I spoke to Roger Short, a scientist working in Australia. He said, emotionally, that the disease was an attack on love itself. And what kind of world was that? He was so furious at the slow progress in reducing new HIV infections that he was looking at any alternative to prevention, especially natural ones that could be freely available to anyone. Truly, "Access for All"! Although he was proposing radical theories of prevention, his ideas were included in that month's issue of the esteemed *Nature* periodical. I'd learn more about his alternatives in the coming months.

I spoke to Steve Wesselingh, another Australian scientist

working on a cutting-edge microbicide, who said, "Basically, entire generations are going to be wiped out unless we take this very seriously."

I got to speak to Mary Robinson, a dignified, charismatic woman. After I posed Kevin's questions to her, I told her how he thought no one understood how he felt.

She agreed, "I don't think we do understand just what it's like to be Kevin and some fourteen million other children who are orphaned by AIDS. How desperate they are. How discriminated against. They're hungry. They are invisible. There's violence against them. And they rightly don't feel that we have given them enough attention. It's part of the problem of trying to put a human face on HIV and AIDS."

"One of the things he said is that basic needs should be met," I said. "He had to sneak into school because of the school fees. Shouldn't he be able to go to school, to eat? These basic needs?"

"He's perfectly right," she responded. "And I would say not even needs. These are his rights. He should be supported because of the fact that he is orphaned by AIDS. And so should all the other children orphaned by AIDS. But there is no doubt whatsoever he is someone whose rights we have guaranteed. His government has guaranteed those rights. The international community has guaranteed those rights. Collectively, states have said it, even if a country's very poor. More than 148 countries have ratified it. Every country, except for the United States and Somalia, has ratified the Convention on the Rights of the Child."

Kevin and I would learn a lot more about his rights later.

I even spoke to a young teenage girl, Kevin's age, from the United States via Nicaragua and Peru: Carolina Réal. Dressed in a tank top and shorts, she told me why she was there, as her younger brother videotaped our videotaping of our interview, and every so often interrupted her as younger brothers do. She had come along to the conference with her mother, who was working for a U.S. broadcaster. She and her brother were going around talking to young people and anyone they could in order to better understand the disease. They'd even met Richard Gere at an orphanage and had their picture taken with him!

Carolina said, "I didn't really think AIDS was a big deal, because I live in a really small town in the United States. We learn about it but it's never really important enough to do anything about it. So I knew it was dangerous. I knew it was out there, but I didn't, really didn't think that I could do anything to help. Until I came here."

I told her about Kevin, and about other children I'd seen in Kenya, Malawi, and now Thailand. She said this: "I think adults just think they know everything. But nothing's being changed. You know, they all talk. And at the conference we're missing a lot of young people. Young people are being infected. Instead of sitting in a session listening to adults speak, I think we should listen to kids speak. And hear their point of view. 'Cause we're the ones that are having the problems."

Each person I met there was passionate. Each had something to offer. But few seemed as affected by the epidemic as Kevin, and I wasn't sure how much they were really offering him in terms of help in their answers. They were coming to his concerns with their own concerns, their own issues—as we all do. After all, we're only human, each seeing the world through our own eyes.

The person I wanted to talk to now was Kevin. I wanted to share what these people had said in response to his questions. To at least show him that, halfway around the world, he had actually been heard. I wanted him to hear especially the sentiment of Sujima, Senator Mechai's daughter who'd championed the cause of young people, ensuring youth were included at events for the first time at the International AIDS Conference. No one, she said, had asked them their ideas on prevention or how to change the course of this disease that would impact them far more than the older leaders here. I had asked her, "If Kevin feels alone, should he? And other orphans? Or are there actually a lot of people around the world their age maybe who do care?"

Sujima had replied, "I hope that this message gets to them: they're not alone. They might feel alone. Their environment might be really harsh to them. But when you reach out your hands, we will touch—somewhere in the moon. But we will touch. I don't know what to say." She almost broke down in tears.

The moon seemed closer than a solution to the epidemic.

CHAPTER SIX
BACK TO KENYA

Five months later, finally, I returned to Kenya. At the time, I was staying in Amsterdam with Sarah, who was workshopping her feature-film project at a prestigious filmmaking program there, but I had become an official resident of Australia. The Australian Film Commission kindly gave Veronica Sive, an Australian producer, and me a loan to shoot the promo—a promo to see if Kevin could hold a film. (Veronica had grown up in South Africa, which had its own severe HIV/AIDS crisis.)

In Nairobi, I stayed overnight with Cathy Scott and her husband, Jim. Cathy Scott is an Australian documentary filmmaker. She and Jim had moved to Nairobi, but we had met at a screening of a film of hers months earlier in Australia. Cathy's dedication to our project—and to Kevin—would prove invaluable, and she worked tirelessly both as director of photography and in securing interviews and researching people.

In their Land Rover, she and I drove from the Kenyan capital, Nairobi, up through the countryside, through the famed Rift Valley, all the way up to Kisumu. I was amazed at just how beautiful the countryside was. On my other recent trips to Africa, I had spent most of my time looking for slums where I would find impoverished and orphaned children, and my first experience of the continent had been the civil war in Sierra Leone! Even so, as we drove through, I was so focused on getting to see Kevin again and getting this film right that I could barely see the beauty around me. It would take more trips for that.

Cathy had been warned that driving on this road at night was not a good idea, that the chances of being robbed were high, so we were trying to make good time. Two muzungus in a Land Rover with a lot of expensive camera gear would make a nice target. But of course Cathy and I couldn't help but get lost and ended up driving in the dark, on potholed roads with not a streetlight in sight. However, after taking endless wrong turns, we finally—hours and hours later—made it to Kisumu. It was too late for us to get a meal, so we went straight to bed in our separate mosquito-netted rooms in the lodging Frederik and Nathalie had organized.

I couldn't sleep. It wasn't the mosquitoes. It wasn't the heat. It wasn't the long drive. It was me.

I was nervous to see Kevin. More nervous than I'd thought I would be. What would he be like after all this time? Perhaps (although I did not realize it at the time) I was more worried than I'd thought about this young person, no longer caring about him just as a filmmaker, but even more as a human being.

The next day, together with Joseph from Pandipieri, who was still counseling Kevin and who had been his conduit to Nathalie and Frederik for his living funds, we drove through the gate into Kisumu Boys School. We told the principal's assistant we were there, and they sent someone to look for Kevin.

I wandered around the hallways looking at this much more grown-up school than where I'd last seen Kevin. A few teachers talked amongst themselves. Young male teenagers in dark red jackets and ties stood around, looking at us. I wandered through hall after hall. After what seemed like eons had passed, someone who looked more like a young man than a boy came walking down the hall. This teenager was Kevin: stronger, more confident than he'd been before, wearing his tie, white shirt, and dark trousers.

And an incredibly huge smile.

I wore a huge smile myself—as if it were stitched to my face. I was ecstatic to see him happy and well.

We hugged.

He was very happy to see me, and I to see him.

We hugged again.

Together, we drove back to the slum, to his shack. It looked the same outside and inside. Green painted door, chipped old mud walls, and he still had as many of his mother's chairs as he'd had before. It was only he who had changed. But he proudly pointed out his new possessions. An alarm-clock radio with a tape player! A calendar.

I gave him some books I'd brought for him, as well as a very childish gift—a big letter K made of chocolate. (He had become fixed in my mind as a twelve-year-old; I find I remember people as I last saw them, not who they've become.)

I also brought a gift from my mother, Chanit. My mother and father both raised me to be who I am, but my mother in particular could relate to Kevin. She had been partially orphaned during World War II, growing up Jewish in what was then Czechoslovakia. Her father had been killed early in the war and, while many of her relatives were murdered, her mother became a partisan, fighting the Nazis from the woods. My mother had been very moved by Kevin's story and wanted him to have a diary to write in.

He was very pleased to have something from her. That seemed to touch a chord in him, and I only realized later how deeply.

We talked about his life. He was still lonely living by himself, but he said he at least had more friends now. Some even visited once in a while. He still cooked for himself, still washed his clothes. He woke up at six o'clock in the morning to make himself breakfast and get himself to school by seven. He stayed at school until six then came home and made himself dinner. He had come fifth in his class the previous semester. He was proud of that!

He studied at night by the light of a paraffin lamp. He confided that sometimes he didn't have the money for paraffin. It was expensive, and he had learned to be "mean," he said, to make the money go further. I hadn't realized that the money we'd organized for him wasn't enough, that he still had to be "mean." What kind of a "mean" fool was I?

Kevin still went to church most Sundays and was a devout Catholic. When I asked him what kind of music he liked listening to, it was the Christian station on the radio that was his favorite. He liked those religious songs. They comforted him. They made him feel less alone.

I reminded him that the last time we'd met he'd wanted to be an AIDS doctor. He said he still did. And so we began to talk about AIDS.

What did he know? What was he being taught? Did he know how he could prevent himself from getting HIV? He was sixteen years old at this point, living in the area that had been worst affected by the epidemic in all of Kenya. If ever someone needed to know how to protect himself from HIV/AIDS, it was Kevin.

It turned out that he didn't know very much. He had been told not to have sex. That many people had AIDS, and that many died, such as his parents. He said he was very scared of AIDS. "I fear it," he said. As the community would grow suspicious if he asked too many questions about it, he had few people he could trust to ask how to keep himself safe. Kevin did trust his next-door neighbor, whom he described as an elder in the community. Kevin went to talk to him sometimes when he was lonely or too tired to cook himself dinner. His name was Albert. We decided to visit Albert together to see what advice he would give Kevin.

CHAPTER SEVEN

ALBERT

Kevin straightened his tie out of respect, getting himself ready, and combed his hair in his little mirror. Then we went to the shack next door. Luckily, Albert was home. He was a "businessman," Kevin said. Many people were businessmen or businesswomen in Kisumu. How else could one get money? Selling something, even tomatoes piled into small pyramids by the side of the road, like many women did, or some old clothes, like men did, meant you had a business and were a businessperson.

Albert, a small man of about forty-five or so, a full head shorter than Kevin, dressed in a green spotted shirt, came out past the crimson gauze cloth hanging down from his doorway. Kevin told him he wanted to ask his advice about AIDS, and Albert invited us in.

It was a small dark room, with a miniature table and two chairs opposite. Newspapers were plastered on the wall as if it were a radical college student's room. But these were simply a form of cheap wallpaper. Some of the stories dated back a few years. One was on Kenyan corruption, another was a picture of a pretty woman with a product, another of 9/11 in New York. Kevin sat with his back to the newspapers, and Albert was somewhat hidden in the darkness, like a much thinner Kurtz from the film *Apocalypse Now*.

Albert had a wife and two children, but the children didn't live with them for some reason that was left unexplained. Kevin and Albert spoke in Swahili, while Joseph translated into English. "I've come to ask you more about HIV/AIDS," Kevin began. "We, as young boys, how do you think we can prevent ourselves from this HIV virus?"

As Kevin listened intently, Albert said, "HIV is recently in existence. If you're not careful, you can easily get it. The first thing to do or remember is your God. You have to go to church. From church, you have to study. After study, you have to go to school. From school, you have to go prepare your food. And if you don't have it, you can come to us. And if you are not in school, remember not to accompany these young girls. For they can easily lead you into temptation. For if you come close to these girls, and you smile at one another, you will be involved in sexual intercourse. And before you decide to be involved in sexual intercourse, don't even think of using these condoms. But pray to your Lord."

Kevin nodded seriously, as I listened, horrified.

Then, not completely understanding Albert's reply, Kevin followed up by asking, "We children with no parents, how can we know that this person or that is not infected? You said that what I need to do is go to church and to school and to house. How can this prevent HIV/AIDS? Can you just see someone and say she is infected?"

Albert continued, kindly but firmly. "AIDS has no age limit. Children and adults can get it. AIDS is even in people with beautiful faces. Because you have no parents, you have to rely on us. You need to understand what we will be telling you. If we tell you this is not good and you go ahead and do it, then you will be doing something almost against your parents. Now that you have come to me, I'm as your parent. If I tell you not to walk with this girl or that, you need to do so. From school to home, to house to school!"

Far away, in Washington, D.C., in the United States, Congress had authorized approximately three billion dollars in HIV-prevention funds to be spent on promoting abstinence until marriage. Much of this money was, at this time, finding its intended way into the hands of evangelical Christian groups, thought best by the current administration to spread the message. (When I'd arrived in Kenya at the airport this time, I had been surprised to hear so many southern accents from the States and see so many groups from different churches.)

Here in Kisumu, Albert repeated himself a few times. In an area of Kenya where 40 percent of the young women Kevin would meet and possibly date would be HIV positive—that is, almost one out of two women—Albert had given Kevin, whose parents had died of HIV/AIDS and who wanted now to know how he could stay alive, this advice: "Don't even think of using these condoms but pray to the Lord."

Kevin had no electricity, no telephone, no Internet access. He could not just Google "AIDS" and find out a different point of view or read about the recommendations of UNAIDS or the World Health Organization.

A telephone call at the call center in town cost ninety-eight shillings a minute to call anywhere outside of Africa. Kevin and most people in his community lived on about seventy-eight shillings a day. It would cost a day's worth of food, clothing, and rent to be put on hold by a computerized answering service at any international organization that might have the answers to Kevin's question of how he and other orphans could protect themselves; a computerized answering service that would most likely not understand his Kenyan accent.

"Don't even think of using these condoms, but pray to the Lord."

When we left the shack, I asked Kevin if he thought this was good advice. He didn't know. I promised him we would work together, do whatever we could, talk to whomever we could, to understand HIV/AIDS, how to prevent it, how to deal with it, and to keep him alive.

Kevin seemed pleased by that.

We shook hands on that promise.

CHAPTER EIGHT

A BRIEF NOTE ABOUT GOD AND CONDOMS

I am no expert on divinity by any means, yet I have made a few documentaries about God—and what we believe about God—in Judaism, in Christianity, in Islam, even Buddhism. I have worked with the World Conference on Religion and Peace. I have worked on stories about Christians and Muslims bringing warring parties to peace talks in Sierra Leone in a horrific civil war. I have been to houses of worship (in the form of churches, synagogues, mosques, or Buddhist temples) in Italy, France, the United Kingdom, the Netherlands, Germany, Switzerland, Britain, the United States, Sierra Leone, Kenya, Malawi, South Africa, Australia, Bhutan, Thailand, Vietnam, and the Philippines.

I have also seen a picture taken by the Hubble Telescope that is the deepest we have ever seen into space. Imagine just your thumb pictured against the night sky. In that picture, which is only about the area of your thumb, there are 750 million galaxies—not stars, but galaxies.

Bearing that in mind, I have a hard time believing that God, him or herself, in whatever form, has really come down against condoms. What I found in trying to answer Kevin's questions was that there were many deeply religious people who agree. Especially given the fact that all religions consider life sacred, and there are some four million new HIV infections every year.

And I am sure we all want Kevin, and all the other deserving children like Kevin, to stay alive. Especially God (I think).

CHAPTER NINE

THE EFFECT OF NO CONDOMS, STIGMA, AND PREPARING TO DIE

Where Kevin lives in Kisumu, approximately one out of four people is HIV positive. But few would admit it.

When I'd first gone there, almost no one would get tested. This is the stigmatization of the disease. There are as many superstitions about AIDS as there are people who are HIV positive. As Kevin, now sixteen years old, said to me when I was trying to get him to acknowledge on camera that his parents had died of AIDS, "If someone's parents have died, he or she cannot just come in public and say my parents died of AIDS. Because he or she will feel ashamed. People think that it is only acquired through prostitution. Now, when someone's open publicly that he is HIV positive, people will think that maybe he or she was a prostitute."

In the "developed" West, there was nothing to crow about in regard to stigmatization, either. I remember in the '80s how a child with AIDS in America, named Ryan, had eventually become a popular hero years after enduring abuse, avoidance, and public battles to keep him in school. Also in America, the disease was stigmatized early on by some who regarded it as God's punishment of homosexuals. Some might even argue that that stigma has clouded the entire AIDS epidemic to date!

The gospel-flavored stigma has continued throughout sub-Saharan Africa. The Kenyan newspapers are full of pictures of young and middle-aged people who are "promoted to glory" or who are "late," but with no mention of what they died of (or were late for). When you do ask someone what their relatives may have died of, the answer is certainly not AIDS.

My friend in Mombasa, Lucy Yinda, a middle-aged, extraordinarily intelligent woman, has a special take on this. Lucy comes from a prominent family. She herself has spent the last ten years focusing on helping street children through an organization she founded called Wema Centre (where Ann the nurse and Evelyn the pilot were from). She has helped about ten thousand children to date.

Lucy told me the story of how she went to a funeral in the "rural areas" of one family member whom everyone knew had died of AIDS. However, at the funeral, all anyone could talk about was the relative's tragic "car crash." Finally, one of her nieces, who worked at the World Bank in Nairobi, cried out, "We all know they didn't die in a car crash! If we can't even admit that our relative died of AIDS, but insist they died in a car crash when they were nowhere near a car, how can we ever stop this epidemic?"

My camerawoman, Cathy Scott; Joseph, Kevin's counselor; Kevin; and I needed to find people locally who were HIV positive themselves, willing to be open and honest about their condition. We needed them for our film, and for Kevin. Kevin was living around so many infected people but all he knew were rumors and innuendo, not an openly HIV-positive person. What was it really like to live with HIV in Kisumu?

Joseph knew someone who would be willing to talk. Her name was Edwina.

Edwina lived in a neighboring slum, and Joseph had been assigned by Pandipieri to counsel her as well. She was twenty-one years old and had a four-year-old son named Fedel. He was going to the nursery school at the Centre. That was where we were going to pick up her and her son and then take her to her home where she and Kevin could speak.

When Albert said AIDS is in people with beautiful faces, he was surely talking about people like Edwina. Dressed in a throwaway white T-shirt and black trousers, she had smooth dark skin, and wide brown eyes that revealed so much love when she stroked the head of her little boy. He was dressed in a red sweater (in the Kisumu heat!) and red shorts, and he just stared at the ground, nodding yes and no when Kevin tried to speak to him, holding onto his mother's hand.

All together, we drove to Edwina's mud shack with a rusted corrugated roof, not dissimilar to Kevin's, but with photographs of her parents on a little table, and a white brocade curtain swinging in the doorway. The place consisted of three small rooms: one tiny waiting room in front, another in the back for her son and herself, and a third for her roommate who shared the costs of the rent. Yes, the rent of the shack.

Kevin was obviously uncomfortable talking to Edwina about HIV at first, but slowly slowly—*polé polé*, as they say in Swahili—he relaxed a little.

Edwina told him she had decided to be brave and come out about her status, but people in her community had not reacted positively, as Kevin had predicted. She said, "First in my family, they discriminated me after discovering my status. But within my community, they, too, know about my status. Because I'm out speaking public about my status. And they know that I'm HIV positive. But being that, they are doing me such bad things, bad habits toward me."

Kevin asked her about when she had found out she had the disease. She told him, "Yes, I know my status. I knew my HIV status in the year 2001."

After a long pause, Kevin continued, "And how were the results and how did you feel about it?"

"It was positive. That means I was HIV infected. I was shocked. But due to how I had been living with a long sickness, I just accepted it. Because I'd really suffered a lot."

"What kind of suffering?" Kevin asked. "Can you tell me?"

"I was first diagnosed with TB. And I was every now and then having malaria that is off and on."

(Tuberculosis and malaria are two diseases that tend to kill a lot of people in sub-Saharan Africa. In fact, sometimes Kevin would say his mother died of malaria. But AIDS weakens the body to the point that people who might otherwise survive are dying of these diseases. In fact, scientists are now investigating whether malaria speeds up the spread of AIDS. But there is no public stigma to dying either of it or TB. The UN and G8 countries created the Global Fund to fight AIDS, Tuberculosis, and Malaria in 2002.)

The next question Kevin asked with some difficulty: "So . . . so can I ask . . . So when you got the result positive, was there any evidence that can show you have to get it, such as you are having unsafe sex, such things?"

"I was once married. But my husband divorced me when I was really sick. But when I married, I got him with three wives. I being the fourth one. So there is where I thought my infections came from."

"So your infection came through your husband."

"The reason why I'm saying that I got infection through marriage is that I was just from school, and I was married off. And he's the only man who started—whom I started friendship with. That means he's the one who infected me."

Her family had married off Edwina, at the age of fifteen, to a man in Tanzania. She was literally his fourth wife. (In many rural areas, polygamy is still practiced.) When she got sick, the husband didn't want to care for her. He wrote a letter to her parents that they should come for her until she got better. Back in Kenya, on her parent's subsistence farm, she was sick, endlessly sick. We saw pictures of her then, bone thin—a sharp contrast to the healthy and wide-cheeked but obviously tired and distressed young woman she was now.

At that time her boy was only two months old. She decided to get an HIV test for herself and her baby. She tested positive;

he negative. She didn't understand how she could be positive and her own son not. But she was grateful for Fedel's results. The most positive thing for her was that, because she had come out publicly, she also managed to get on a government trial program for antiretroviral drugs. These drugs were at that point very difficult to get in Kenya or anywhere in sub-Saharan Africa, but had been keeping people in the developed world alive since the mid-'90s.

When her husband found out her status, even though she was now well enough to go back to him, he told her parents that he didn't want either her or her son. He'd already married another fourth wife, "who was more special for him," said Edwina, shrugging.

Living with her parents in a small village not far from Kisumu was not easy, either. Edwina's mother accused her of bringing shame on the family.

So she moved to Kisumu to this shack that she and her son shared with her friend. She had always wished to work in an office but, after her illness and having left school early, she knew she wouldn't be able to go to college. So she began to be a "businesswoman" and, feeling she had nothing to be ashamed of, she told people here as well that she was HIV positive.

"When I started selling things like sukamaweeki, green vegetables, things like chips, they would not buy them. If they saw some neighbors buying them, the person buying could be ashamed and told, "Why are you . . . why are you buying some AIDS things? Are you ready to get AIDS?" So after hearing all this I felt so bad because of their bad attitudes to me. For I know that even if I sell something, I don't infect somebody. But they believe that I can infect them by giving them or selling them something. And they continue pointing at me and saying, 'You see this girl, she's this,' whenever I worked."

Unable to sell food or vegetables, she talked with a job counselor from the Centre. He suggested that maybe if she sold things that people didn't eat, they wouldn't be afraid of getting AIDS. So she sold charcoal. After all, how could anyone get HIV from charcoal? At least this way she managed to meet her basic needs.

She desired one day to get a little plot of land that she could raise her son on to build a "happy happy home," but she had no idea how to go about doing this and wished the government could somehow help her.

Even on medication, Edwina knew she faced her own mortality—at the age of twenty-one. Because of that, she was writing a "memory book" to leave for her son. In it, she pasted pictures of herself, pictures of him, and wrote little memories and anecdotes. The book, like a photo album, began with a picture of Fedel, and the inscription "This book is for you" written by Edwina.

Kevin, always the intense boy, asked her about her death straight on. "Are you worried upon your death how Fedel will continue with life without you?" And then again, as if this were a normal conversation between sixteen- and twenty-one-year-olds, "Are you frightened about death?"

"I'm not worried about death," Edwina replied, "because I know that death is there. Somebody is born to live and after all die. The only thing that I'm fighting for is how I can leave my only son. To try and write for him a memory book to understand who his mum was, and how his family was broken up. And if indeed I could have land, I could let him know that through writing a memory book. Meaning that anything that is belonging to me, my only son could inherit. Nobody could take it in my absence, because it will be recorded in my memory book that I'm already writing. That's why everything, everything that I, his mum, wanted him to have, I'm putting them in a memory book. At least my child, I could leave him with everything written."

When Kevin asked what could be done to prevent HIV/AIDS in young people like him, Edwina said she hoped the government would spread the truth about prevention. And that girls wouldn't be forced by their families to marry so young, as she had been. She didn't have advice for Kevin but rather for the girls—the girls her age in Kisumu, 40 percent of whom, as mentioned earlier, were HIV positive but couldn't admit it. "If it is a matter of marriage, don't just go about marriage. Know about your partner's HIV status first, and then have a healthy marriage. And, for girls, don't allow your parents to marry you off the way I was married off. Because it is you and you alone that will bear the downs."

Yet this young woman, whose community would not buy vegetables because of the stigma attached to her, whose own family had discriminated against her, was trying to help this community. A few times a week, she spoke at the local district hospital to groups of pregnant women. She explained how they could prevent mother-to-child transmission of the virus, told them about the drugs they could take, and urged them to go and get tested for HIV. Otherwise, she emphasized, they could be condemning themselves and their children.

We went to see her there, in a small antiseptic room. She spoke honestly about herself and her child, and I watched the women listen intently, taking her so much more seriously than any nurse, doctor, or foreign charity worker. This woman who had been made an outcast by her own village was overcoming any feelings of anger and bitterness she might have. Worried for her own life and that of her son, Edwina was still doing whatever she possibly could with the little she had to prevent her fate from happening to others.

I didn't fully realize it at the time, but Kevin and I had just had the privilege of getting to know a hero.

CHAPTER TEN
MEMORY BOOKS

Kevin was impressed by the idea of a memory book. It was something he mulled over as we drove back to his shack, something he mulled over for days. His mother had not left him a memory book; she'd left him nothing but those photographs he found difficult to look at and her chairs that he refused to sell.

The concept of memory books is becoming widespread throughout Africa. They create a connection from generation to generation, a connection that otherwise could disappear, particularly if a child was taken out of the community. Beyond sharing the story of the parents, the memory book can also lay out for the child what the family properties are, in the hope that relatives and others won't steal them. It is a legacy for the child, so that they are not left rootless like Kevin.

The famous Swedish crime novelist Henning Mankell (also an AIDS activist) wrote his own touching book on his experiences in Uganda concerning memory books. He claimed memory books could form a new "library of Alexandria"—where the memories of millions of people will be collected; that their contents will be what is remembered of our lives.

At the very least, they are a way of keeping some continuity and letting Kevin's entire generation have some link with their past, a past that previously had been passed down mainly orally. (How many of us know almost nothing of our backgrounds, our parents or grandparents, even without being impacted by AIDS?)

Edwina's book for her boy, Fedel, at the very least would allow her to share her memories of her grandparents, parents, and her life with him, as well as her memories of her love and life with her boy. Her twenty-one-year-old life.

CHAPTER ELEVEN

DEATH AND WATERGATE

As I've mentioned, I had seen someone at the dying stage—emaciated, delirious—in 2001, not long after first meeting Kevin. This was a man named Joseph Musyoka. He had once been a proud and strong human being, a family man, an educated man, with a construction business in central Kenya. When I met him through a referral from a nurse at Mombasa's public hospital, he could walk only with the help of his son and his wife, Jane (also HIV positive and, as she said, infected by him). She was an amazingly strong yet openly emotional woman, pouring out her own grief and worry. The son was fourteen, distraught to see his father so sick. His name was Nixon, named for the American president Richard Nixon, who had resigned from office in the midst of scandal, but a man whom Joseph had much admired.

They were living in Joseph's family compound, a decently

constructed group of cement dwellings around a small court-yard in the midst of a slum of absolute squalor. One sees quite a few of these in Africa. Desperate for places to live, people settle or squat on government land, building shantytowns. When some people prosper, instead of buying land, they just build better houses in their midst.

I sat talking with the Musyokas first in the small courtyard; I was with my taxi driver, a devout Muslim. He became the sound person for this interview, as Christian was off filming elsewhere. A strong man, he was deeply shaken by the story of Joseph and Jane, who could openly cry in front of complete strangers. Nixon himself could barely speak—or cry. His emotions were literally choking him.

Joseph said he'd got HIV from a "car crash," but Jane later confided she did not believe him. He said when they had come back to Mombasa to live at the family compound, his parents refused to let them eat with them in the main house. Instead they all had to share one room on the side. Joseph had brought shame on the family, having come back home to die with this sickness, disgraced like that president he'd admired.

I gave them $100. This was not enough for medicine, but I thought that it would be a bit of help. As far as I knew at this time, antiretroviral drugs were barely available in Kenya.

When I returned to follow up two months later, this time with Christian, Joseph was on his deathbed. He was speaking deliriously to his son, spittle foaming in his mouth. Jane was much thinner, too, but not like her husband. He was only skin and bone, reminding me of the pictures of Holocaust survivors.

Jane said it was difficult to care for him. He was dying, but it was for the best. This way they could get on with their lives: Nixon with his school, and Jane with her need to make a living.

My last memory of those three that day is of Jane sitting sewing, Nixon sitting on his father's bed, and Joseph barely able to raise his head, whispering incoherently and painfully, trying to say something to his son.

I learned later from Jane that Joseph died the next day.

When speaking about this disease, I want this to be clear: I have no right to feel or act self-righteous. I could have provided more money to Joseph Musyoka to enable him to stay alive, to get medicines, to get healthy so he could provide for his family. Had I really researched whether there were medicines he could take?

It's not that simple.

But . . .

I could have done more. I didn't.

Joseph Musyoka still haunts me. I still see him, eyes too wide for their sockets, calling out to his son. He could have acquired HIV from a car crash and blood transfusion, as he claimed. Or from sex with someone other than Jane, as she told me later she was sure was the case.

But most of the world does not believe in death for adulterers. Is death by HIV/AIDS then all right?

Jane Musyoka wanted to start a home-based care program to help other HIV sufferers. Keri Douglas, who'd arranged the screening of *14 Million Dreams* at the National Press Club and the charity event, organized monies for her.

Jane became an advocate. She appeared in an article in the national newspaper, which she e-mailed to me. She spoke at a conference in front of national religious leaders and international figures from UNICEF and the UN. A friend of mine who'd been at the conference told me that she had praised me for finding her family and taking care of them. Considering I felt completely as if I'd done otherwise, I was moved.

Jane died last year. Another hero.

Her children are orphaned now, too. I don't know if she wrote a memory book for them, or if the enduring image she might have left them is her crying in our film.

Chapter Twelve

Jane Ochola and God

Kevin did get to meet a different Jane: Jane Ochola. Jane had four children. Both she and her husband, Peter, were HIV positive and admitted it. Jane, however, was very sick and had full-blown AIDS.

Cathy had badly injured her ankle in one of the infamous street holes of Kisumu the night before, so it was just Joseph, Kevin, and me. As we walked toward Jane's shack, Joseph confided quietly that basically she was very close to dying.

We first sat with Peter in the front room, separated from Jane by a hanging cloth and the mud wall. Peter sat with his back against the window, the curtain rising and falling with the breeze to let in the light or keep us in darkness. He spoke about his fears of raising the children alone. He had a job working at the church, but it didn't pay much. A good portion of their money was going to care for his wife now. Medicines for her were difficult to get. His condition was somehow easier. He wasn't self-pitying; he spoke matter-of-factly, softly. Kevin didn't find it difficult to talk to him and ask questions, but he didn't ask Peter if he'd given his wife HIV.

I went into the other room to speak with Jane before Kevin came in. She lay prone on a slim mattress on the floor. She was skin and bone, a beautiful woman perhaps in her late thirties (it was hard to tell), wasting away. Her eyes were strong, white, haunted. I explained why we were there and asked whether that was all right. She nodded.

Then Kevin came in quietly, pushing past the dark cloth, to sit opposite her. He nodded and said, "Jambo." She whispered, "Jambo" back. And then he sat still.

For many minutes he could not or would not speak.

He looked away from her. He looked straight ahead or at the window, with this curtain, too, rising and falling in eerie soft gusts to let in either blinding light or nothing at all.

I studied her long thin fingers, the gaunt cheekbones protruding in her face. Maybe I was trying to find Joseph Musyoka in her.

I wondered if I was being irresponsible in letting Kevin see Jane. She could only have reminded him of his mother. Did he need reminding? Who was I to come here and do this to a boy who had already suffered so much?

But here we were. I prodded him, whispered to him to speak, as did Joseph, who held the microphone.

Jane finally raised herself so that she was leaning her head on her elbow, looking straight at Kevin.

Finally Kevin spoke to her. "How do you feel?"

She just coughed.

"When did the disease start?"

"It's about three years now."

"When it started, what was your first step?" he asked. "Do you normally use medicine even if you are not sick?"

"Yes. I use antibiotics and multivitamins."

Kevin nodded in all seriousness. At this point, he didn't understand about medicines specifically for this disease Jane had, only having briefly heard about antiretrovirals from Edwina.

"You have children," he said quietly. "How do you feel about their future?"

Jane spoke, looking straight at him. "I don't think much about it. Because if I think about it, it gives me a lot of stress and worry. I leave it in the hands of God."

Kevin now looked down and a look of gentle vulnerability came over his face. "Even now as you are seeing me, I'm an orphan. My parents died of HIV [he admitted the letters HIV to her] and life has been difficult. And I'd also like to encourage you to talk with your children. That even if God takes you away, life has to continue, as I'm also facing the same."

She coughed again and spoke gently. "That's why I don't want to think about my children's future. Because if I do so, it will give me so many troubles. I've left everything in the hands of God. Who knows what He will have to do with the children? We can't say we live forever. But it's Him who knows what will happen with the children."

Later, her children came in to be with her. The littlest boy sat on his brother's lap, who sat on the mattress beside Jane. She looked at them with evident and deep-welled love. The older brother dipped the little boy's cap, causing him to giggle with the delight only a little child can muster at such a simple sign of affection.

By the window, her eldest daughter, a teenager, stared down at her mother, then at the wall, as Kevin had done. Silently. Kevin and she now both stared at the same spot on the mud wall, as the curtain rose and fell, now blindingly light, now dark as death.

We took our leave and walked outside. It was a beautiful day. We passed busy chickens, and men working on furniture outside. We went to Lake Victoria, looking out over the painted fishing boats, men reeling in their large nets.

Kevin didn't say anything. I didn't say anything.

Joseph and I drove him back to his hut. We were going to drop him by the road right near his shack, leaving him to walk home from there. Normally, he didn't want us to come into the slum, thinking we, and he, would receive too much unwanted attention from some of the unemployed young men hanging around by the stalls.

This time, however, he asked me to come with him.

We went to his hut. He showed me his clock radio again. He showed me the calendar again. We sat and talked about everything except what had happened this afternoon with Jane. We just quietly enjoyed our company together.

I thought Kevin, after having now spoken to people living

with AIDS, needed to hear about more than not using condoms and God's wishes. Or, if God did have wishes, what did He or She wish for Kevin and the millions of children like him?

CHAPTER THIRTEEN
CHILDREN

What the children I've spoken to wish for is to go to school. They adore it. In the crowded classrooms, if a teacher asks a question, their hands shoot up immediately. It feels as if you're in a forest of hands, all straining for the teacher's, the sun's, attention.

When the children take a break from the crowded hot classrooms, they play madly in the yard. Many of the schools have old painted ads for Coca Cola on the walls, which you see behind the kids kicking soccer balls or playing jump rope.

Some of the uniforms consist of green sweaters, ties, white shirts, and shorts. Others have blue sweaters. Valentine's was a blue sweater and yellow skirt. Some girls have red skirts. And these children keep their clothes clean. When I show people in Australia or America photographs, one of the things everyone is always impressed by is how clean the students' white shirts are. How do they keep their white shirts so white?, people ask.

I'd always been impressed with Kevin, too, in that regard, just how clean he kept his clothes, washing them in the washbasin. Though the shirt was old and worn at the collar when I first met him, it was spotless. And I saw how his neighbor, Albert's wife, washed endlessly, with pride, as if that itself would keep poverty at bay.

The younger children play with whatever toys they can find. Bicycle tires are popular; kids push them along with a stick for hours. At nursery schools (such as the one Edwina's son, Fedel, attended), kids take great pleasure calling out to an adult like myself wandering by. "HOW ARE YOU?" the children will scream with delight.

"I'm fine," I reply. (I lie, as an adult!) "How are you?" And you really want them to tell you how they are.

"HOW ARE YOU?" the children scream again in reply.

Then there are others. These kids live on the streets of Kisumu, begging on the main thoroughfare. They wear old T-shirts. They sniff glue and squabble over bread if you buy it for them. Their fighting can get intense. They have so little. The small ones want to eat. The big ones want to eat.

They seem to have become used to living on the street or sniffing glue, these ones—like Ann Njeri and Evelyn had before being rescued by Lucy Yinda.

Many, however, want to go to school. (Kevin and I would meet some of these together.) But even though the law has now changed in Kenya, and primary school is finally free, they don't. Most cannot.

As one government official told me, "When we made school

free, all these parents sent their kids to school. There were over a million new students now. But no new teachers. No new desks. Few new schools."

That was the situation for the children with parents. Not street kids. If they could go to school, where would they do their homework? By the light of the moon?

There is a moon shining over the Pacific Ocean tonight where I sit writing, creating a path across the water. It's so strong a ray of light that it looks like one could walk across it and up into the moon itself. I imagine all the millions of children dropping their bottles of glue and walking across the water.

But that's a fantasy.

Reality is something I heard at the AIDS Conference in a study presented by the Nelson Mandela Foundation: the longer children attended school, the better their chances were of preventing HIV infection. Yet secondary school costs so much.

The reality is that children are vulnerable, easily victimized. In societies that have so little, they are the easiest targets. And orphans, with no parents to protect them, are even easier to prey on, and more prone to being infected. Girls are forced into sex at very young ages, as are boys. Or they're seduced by the promise of a meal.

Reality also hit over Christmas when Kevin finally went to see his uncle up in Eldoret, a bus trip of four hours away. Although he left his shack for just a few days, he was robbed. The thieves took his alarm-clock radio. They took some schoolbooks. They took the diary my mother had given him. Nathalie e-mailed me and told me Kevin was especially upset about that.

Later, another adult in the community, someone who'd been trusted by Nathalie, Frederik, and me to deliver money to Kevin, stole from the envelope the monies intended for Kevin to live on. The person unwittingly left the letter telling Kevin there was some money in the envelope, which was how he realized he'd been robbed by adults yet again.

For Kevin, adults not only died on you, but they were also hard to trust. Yet Kevin desperately needed to find adults with information he could trust, in order to keep himself alive. That was part of our journey to come.

CHAPTER FOURTEEN

SCIENCE AND CONDOMS

As part of Kevin's next step, we went to speak to Monica Nyambaka, the nurse at the local Voluntary Counseling and Testing Centre at Pandipieri. The clinic was crowded with people waiting to see the nurses: families, young men, middle-aged men and women. All sitting silently, just waiting.

We went into Monica's small examining room, and, dressed in her white lab coat, she motioned for Kevin to jump up and sit on the green bed. He asked her about the epidemic.

Monica told Kevin that even their health workers were dying of HIV/AIDS. "HIV can affect anybody," she told him.

He seemed very innocent as he asked her if there was a cure. He must know there is no cure, I thought. That was also what Monica told him. "There is no cure. We have what we call antiretrovirals, which can treat this disease and help people live longer."

Kevin parroted some figures he'd heard from a conversation between Nathalie and myself the previous day about half of the women ages eighteen to thirty-four being positive, and male youths between fifteen and twenty-four—trying to appear more informed than he was. He asked what Monica was "telling the youth."

She said, "We have what we call safe sex, which we discuss with the youth. We also teach about abstinence . . . but of course people find it very difficult." She explained more about safe sex, that it necessitated the use of condoms. Kevin just stared at her, perhaps remembering what he'd heard from Albert: no matter what, do not use a condom but pray to the Lord.

She asked him, as she knew his story, if he knew why his parents had died. He smiled.

"Yes."

She asked him if he could tell her.

Kevin then lied and, looking down, told her he didn't know.

"You don't know what your parents died of?" she asked.

"No," he lied.

Even though he knew she knew, he would not tell her. Kevin could not even tell the nurse. Perhaps because she, too, was an adult.

The big question was whether Monica was right. Were condoms the only way, particularly given that Kevin had heard that "God" was against them? We needed to find out what the current scientific truths were.

In Kisumu, a massive study was taking place to see whether circumcision could prevent the transmission of HIV/AIDS.

More than five thousand young men were being circumcised, in a trial organized by Robert Bailey, an anthropologist from the University of Chicago. He turned out to be a friend of Nathalie's, as well as connected to several other people I knew, such as Roger Short, the reproductive biology scientist I'd met at the AIDS Conference who'd been promoting cheap alternative methods of prevention, such as the lemon juice idea.

Kevin met with Robert outside his UNIM (Universities of Nairobi, Illinois, and Manitoba) clinic and laboratory. The two then walked through the crowd of young men all sitting waiting to be tested for HIV and/or circumcised.

In the privacy of his office, Robert explained to Kevin that people from the Luo tribe, the dominant tribe in the area, didn't get circumcised. (Only around 10 percent of Luo men are circumcised. Kevin was of the Luya tribe, of which 85 percent do get circumcised.) In Kisumu, Robert confirmed to Kevin, the AIDS epidemic was the worst of anywhere in Kenya. Approximately 22 percent of the general population was HIV positive.

Yet in areas where people were ritually circumcised, such as in West Africa, the AIDS epidemic infection rate was only 5 to 7 percent. This was even though many of the other conditions were the same, such as poverty, location on trucking routes, prostitution, etc. Though the circumstantial evidence that circumcision could be effective was impressive, many people were not convinced. That was why Robert and his team were carrying out this study right here in Kevin's hometown, funded by the United States National Institute of Health. Another major study was taking place in South Africa.

Kevin wanted to know whether, if circumcision turned out to work, that meant one didn't have to use condoms.

Robert's answer was no. It offered better protection than nothing (seven times better it seemed, mind you), but he would still insist that men use condoms.

Kevin nodded. He was obviously not convinced, although he liked wandering around the laboratory and watching everyone in their white coats.

Then Kevin asked, thoughtfully, "What about women?" What was there for women? Robert replied that Roger Short and other scientists were studying ways women could possibly protect themselves. And one place they were undertaking this research was in Australia.

CHAPTER FIFTEEN
FROM BOTSWANA TO AUSTRALIA

It was our good fortune that Anna Laffy, who'd edited *14 Million Dreams* and become attached to Kevin as a result of watching him over and over again, had moved back to Australia. She had her own child now, but she wanted to work with us on the new film. Being an excellent researcher and former nurse herself, she set up the Australian part of the story.

One of the conceits of this film was that I would not do the interviews, but rather that young people like Kevin would do them. After all, as Carolina had said, it was their generation that was being affected. These young people could confront the experts with Kevin's concerns much more directly, and hopefully gain more than pat answers—as his life was depending on what they found out.

Through Roger Short, Anna enlisted two medical students (as Kevin hoped to be one day) to work with us. They were from

Botswana, now internationally famous for the "No. 1 Ladies Detective" series of books as well as the beautiful Okavango Delta. Though one of the most affluent and stable countries on the African continent, Botswana had an adult HIV prevalence rate of 37 percent. The two students were Max, a thin, handsome young man with a goatee, in his midtwenties, and Sennye, a strong, attractive woman a few years younger. They were on a government grant from Botswana—as the country needed all the doctors it could get and had no medical schools—and attending Melbourne University. With such a high infection rate in their own country, they could understand Kevin's concerns. And Sennye was worried about how women could protect themselves.

When we met on the large campus, we sat on the steps outside one of the older stone buildings and talked about the epidemic and its effect on them. Sennye said she was now twenty-two and, because of HIV/AIDS, life expectancy in Botswana had dropped from seventy to thirty-six years of age. So, technically, she was "more than halfway dead."

Max understood Kevin's reluctance to tell Monica, the nurse, how his parents had died, given all the stigma attached to the disease. Max's mother had died when he was fourteen. When he and I met, it was just after Nelson Mandela had finally publicly acknowledged that his own son had died of HIV/AIDS. Max said, "Of course he can come out and acknowledge that. He is a world-famous figure, the former president of South Africa, and a leader against apartheid. And look how long it took him."

Max continued that, though Nelson Mandela might be praised for coming out about his son, the consequences for Kevin or Max would be the opposite. They would face discrimination and ostracism.

Max and Sennye had started an organization called BAM (Botswana AIDS Melbourne) to organize the approximately one hundred Botswanans now studying there into figuring out AIDS prevention strategies for when they went home. When I met these two, they were busy organizing their first ball.

Both felt like outsiders in Australia, a primarily white country with a sizeable Asian population. There were positive differences between home and Melbourne—in terms of the variety of foods, a wonderful range from Greek to Thai. (As they pointed out, there was still no McDonald's in Gabarone, the Botswanan capital.) There were similarities, too. As we stood among a large group of students being served burgers and beer, singing a drinking song, I thought about Max telling me about Christmas in Botswana: "Party!"

But they said no one in Melbourne could understand what it was like to grow up where they did, because of the epidemic. For example, Sennye pointed out that students on campus could not understand how just dating someone back home could be a life-threatening experience. They couldn't understand what it was like to be told "ABC" (Abstain, Be faithful, Condomize) from the age of ten. And yet Australians also didn't understand how traditionally conservative a culture Botswana was sexually. Sennye could not speak to her mother about sex, or even that she might have a boyfriend. So, she said, many girls, for example, would have multiple boyfriends instead, putting themselves at greater risk.

Max's mentor at the university was Roger Short.

Born in the United Kingdom but now living in Australia, Roger was a charismatic man now in his seventies with a very strong background in reproductive biology but now working somewhat outside the mainstream of science. He also had a great love of Africa, having first been to Kenya in 1962. He'd had a lifelong interest in and commitment to family planning, spending a year working with the WHO in Geneva on HIV/AIDS prevention in 1989.

Now working out of Melbourne University in a small, extraordinarily (and proudly) cluttered office, Short was convinced that the only way to stop the epidemic in Africa was through the use of low-cost prevention methods, which no one I'd met disagreed with. Where he differed were in his ideas for prevention. He said that, although condoms might work elsewhere, perhaps in Thailand, they were obviously not working in Africa, and thus he was promoting the idea of circumcision for Africa even before the final results were in.

He had befriended Max, and the student was impressed by the idea of circumcision as prevention and was researching it intensely himself. Short had encouraged him to learn the low-cost Plastibel technique of circumcision, with Max even making a video that he could then show—and did show later—to doctors and nurses back home in Botswana.

But for women, Roger told both Sennye and Max, his real hope was lemon juice: lemon juice as a microbicide. Microbicides had recently been talked about in the scientific community as the most important new prevention possibility on the horizon. As mentioned earlier, it was hoped that a vaccine against AIDS could be found. But as trial after trial failed to show protection against the virus, it was believed now, in 2005, that a vaccine was at least five to ten years away. Meanwhile, women were becoming the majority victims of the epidemic, women like Edwina or Jane Musyoka, infected by HIV-positive husbands.

To protect herself, a woman could insert a microbicide in the form of a gel (or liquid) prior to having sex, where it would then kill off the HIV virus in any sperm that entered her. However, Roger Short believed that conventional science and big pharmaceutical and biotech companies, in it for profit, were taking far too long to develop these microbicides, while thousands of women were being infected daily. For him, there was enough primary evidence to show that lemon juice itself would work. In Nigeria, there were prostitutes who'd been safely douching with lemon juice for years and weren't HIV positive. In the lab, Roger had tested a concentration of lemon juice, and it had killed most of the HIV virus in about two minutes. Roger's argument was that you could buy five lemons in Kenya for the price of one condom, and the amount of juice from one lemon could be enough for three or four uses.

However, other scientists were not convinced. Scientists such as Dr. David Cooper and Dr. Sean Emery at the National Centre for HIV Epidemiology at the University of New South Wales in Sydney. There had been no scientifically run safety studies in human beings. Though Roger and his colleague in Thailand, Senator Mechai, who hosted the AIDS Conference and whom I'd meet again later, had said they were going to run a safety trial back in July 2004—a safety trial of just fourteen women—as of September 2005 that had still not begun. (Much to Short's and Mechai's consternation, to be fair.)

Dr. Emery pointed out that, considering the amount of misinformation in Africa and the reluctance of everyone to use condoms anyway, promoting lemon juice when it had not been proven was not sound science. Perhaps it might worsen abrasions or cuts, allowing women to be in fact more easily infected with the HIV virus.

Talking with Sennye in the bare kitchen at Max's house, she made it clear she didn't believe that women would use a lemon and "stick it up their vagina. A lemon is a fruit."

She proved that by cutting a lemon in half at the kitchen table. She said that she actually liked lemons, as sour as they were, and put the lemon wedge in her mouth, smiling.

It was Max who made the sour face, not her. She just ate the lemon with pleasure.

On the trail of microbicides, Max and Sennye met with Steve Wesselingh at the Burnet Institute. I'd met Steve at the AIDS Conference, too. He was the one who'd warned about the danger of "an entire generation being wiped out."

A nonprofit organization that worked in virology and populations mainly in Southeast Asia and the Pacific, the Burnet Institute was also concerned about the AIDS epidemic exploding in Papua New Guinea, right next door to Australia.

In partnership with a private company called Starpharma, they had developed a microbicide that was now going into safety trials. The partnership with Starpharma was somewhat of a novelty, a combination of a commercial biotech company and an NGO. The idea behind it was to keep the price of the gel down and have it sold at cost in the developing world (paid for by NGOs, UN agencies, and/or governments) and only make profits for the commercial company in the developed world.

In the labs, Steve explained to Sennye and Max how their microbicide would work—which they understood far better than I did—showing them slides of the "dendrimer-based nanotechnology." When Max asked how far away it was, Steve said he was confident that, within a few years, the Burnet Institute/Starpharma microbicide would be available on a wide scale. And they were at the forefront of microbicide research, funded by the U.S. National Institute of Health, along with some companies in the United States.

When Steve asked Sennye what she thought, she told him honestly that if a bunch of white men came to Botswana and told women there what to put inside their vaginas, women would not use it. Steve agreed. They would have to get the local communities on board.

When Max asked whether microbicides alone would work or if women would still need to use condoms, Steve did acknowledge that they would still encourage women even with the microbicide to use a condom.

And as far as Kevin was concerned, realistically, Steve said, at the moment, with what we had now—and considering the evidence of even the circumcision studies to date—the best prevention was . . . condoms.

Later on, back in Max's house, Sennye made her main argument. (After Max had received high marks for his thesis on circumcision, incidentally!) The point was, she said, condoms worked. So why spend all this time looking at other things when condoms worked?

And, as far as she was concerned, all this telling people about abstinence was rubbish. Abstinence was unrealistic. "Be faithful" to whom? Serial monogamy meant that, even if you were faithful to someone you went out with for six months, you would both go out with someone after the relationship ended, and so the possibilities for infection multiplied. Sennye felt it was most important to push what worked. . . .

Condoms.

CHAPTER SIXTEEN
CONDOMS, CONDOMS, CONDOMS

When I showed Kevin the footage and photos of Max and Sennye and everything they'd seen and discussed, he said that he would abstain from sex. That would work. I tried to point out that, as Monica the nurse had said, he might find that difficult. He insisted he would abstain, period, until he got married. The condom message was still not getting through. The myths and rumors in Kisumu were too widespread, even for Kevin who had me giving him more facts than most people in his community would have access to.

As it was clear that Kevin liked science, both from his studies and from his curiosity at Bailey's lab, I needed to show Kevin the efficacy of condoms scientifically. Anna and Veronica, the producer, had earlier had an idea for where I should film, so now I showed Kevin my footage of—a condom-testing facility! Run by a company named Enersol started by John Gerofi in

Sydney, Australia, it tested condoms for companies and organizations all over the world, including the United Nations Population Foundation (UNFPA). Gerofi had become involved in safe sex back in the 1970s and had been an early board member of the International Standards Committee advising on condom safety, which became ever more necessary as the AIDS epidemic wreaked havoc.

From the outside, the laboratory seemed almost like a normal house in the leafy suburb of Annandale, maybe twenty minutes from the center of Sydney. Inside, however, on the top floor, were the offices, and downstairs were the various testing facilities.

Of course, condom testing does not involve a bunch of men sitting around in a room putting condoms on.

I saw three kinds of tests. On condom packages, one sometimes sees the words "electronically tested." Enersol had designed one such electronic test that worked like this. Condoms were attached by a lab technician to what were basically electronically connected metal teats. These were connected to a computer, and the condoms were filled with water. The water-filled condoms were then lowered into a bath of water with an electric current running through it.

If the condoms had a hole in them big enough for water to get through, an electric current would go through to the "teat" alerting the computer. And the machine would be marked red. "A water molecule is thousands of times smaller than the HIV virus, so it will pass through a condom much more easily than the virus, any virus," John said. I watched this test over and over again. John even put holes in condoms to show me how the test worked. The machine did in fact detect the electronic transmission and stopped.

Another, simpler, condom-testing method was for laboratory workers to fill condoms with water (they were filled on a rotating device), and then take the condom and roll it on green paper. If there was a leak, one would see the water droplet appear on the paper. Ironically, instead of men doing condom testing, it was predominantly women! There was something decidedly odd about watching women rolling water-filled condoms around.

The most spectacular condom-testing method was in the last room. This room was filled with about twenty pressure testers, all behind strong plastic windows. A condom was wrapped around a perpendicular black tube like object. This was attached to a computer. The tube would pump air into the condom, expanding it like a balloon. The computer would measure the pressure. The tube would keep pumping air, until the condom grew to about just under a meter long, at which point it burst.

I will admit I have not seen many men's erect penises but I do doubt, as did John Gerofi, that there is a man on earth who gets as big or bigger than that!

Later, Gerofi blew up a condom into a balloon and tossed it around the room. He'd told me he has a two-year-old son. I wondered if they played with these balloons.

I asked Gerofi what the ratio was of breakage or condoms that failed, leaked, etc. The official acceptable rate was about 1 in 400. But he said most decent condoms were 1 in 1000. And that again was leakage of water, not HIV. Studies showed that if couples, one of whom was HIV positive and the other negative, used condoms, their status would remain unchanged.

Gerofi believed that if people actually would use condoms, the AIDS epidemic could be eradicated. "At the end of the day," he said, "condoms are the most reliable form of prevention for people who are sexually active. If everybody in Africa used condoms in any situation where they were having unsafe sex, the epidemic would stop."

Even a study by the United States National Institute of Allergy and Infectious Diseases stated that the efficacy of condoms in an ideal situation is 100 percent. The way people actually use them brings the effectiveness down to 85 percent.

Let's return to circumcision and microbicides. In the circumcision study in South Africa, circumcised men were 63 percent less likely than uncircumcised men to get HIV from an HIV-positive woman. Other studies show that it's two to nine times less likely. These are significant numbers, and public health experts are seriously investigating circumcision. However, there are issues involved in going about and circumcising whole populations that are poor and living in hazardous health conditions themselves.

Because of one simple fact, the use of microbicides will be problematic for the Catholic Church and various other religious groups. Like condoms, in most cases, the microbicide will prevent conception, as most microbicides also act as spermicidal agents.

Today, the condom is scientifically proven to be the best method to prevent HIV/AIDS. And yet, according to the UNFPA, for whom John Gerofi tests condoms, total monies by donor countries to buy condoms in 2003 was the equivalent of one condom per man per year in the developing world. How many men are having sex only once a year? Or women? And, according to the UNFPA, young people under the age of twenty-five make up almost a quarter of all people living with HIV. Half of all new HIV cases are among young people aged fifteen to twenty-four; six thousand are infected every day.

Kevin had now turned seventeen.

Dr. Sean Emery said something to me that I wanted to remember. While the crisis provokes serious conflict between those who advocate abstinence versus condoms, religious groups on the right as opposed to religious groups on the left, etc., Emery pointed out that, in this fight, "the enemy is the virus."

The enemy is the virus.

Chapter Seventeen

You've Got to Take Your Tea with Sugar

The question Kevin had was, if condoms did work, were people where he lived using them? What were other people around him recommending? What were men doing? Were they abstaining?

Cathy Scott went up to visit Kevin, while I fiddled around trying to raise more funding to make the film. Together, Cathy and Kevin went around his neighborhood asking people in his slum his questions.

Against a background of food stalls with the corrugated tin roofs, one man, wearing a bright yellow hat, identified himself as Brother Frederick. He explained that safe sex was only for married people. Having sex outside of marriage is "an abomination against God," he said. Condoms were not the answer. "You can see them everywhere," and he pointed around him, "just lying on the streets." People were just using them and throwing them everywhere, and still there was this "scourge." (Later, Cathy and I tried to find condom-strewn streets to film to illustrate his point. No luck.)

Another young man, who said his name was Joseph, explained that he didn't need condoms because he had mainly been faithful with the same girl. Kevin asked him if he was having safe sex. He smiled, took a moment, and said he had not been using the condoms.

Kevin spoke to his male friends at school. Dressed in their red suits and ties, they explained that the epidemic was a terrible thing. But they were going to abstain. They did not have girlfriends now, so they did not need condoms. However, they all seemed to know of "friends" who did have girlfriends, and didn't think they always practiced safe sex.

Kevin spoke to three young women. He asked them if they were under pressure from young men to have sex. The answer to that was obvious. He asked if the men would wear condoms. One of the women replied, "A man will tell you that if you do it . . . if you do it with a condom, he will not get that pleasure. He will tell you that sex with a condom is like tea without sugar. We have to take this tea with sugar."

In the worst-hit, AIDS-ravaged area in Kenya, people wanted more sugar for their tea?

Kevin needed to speak to someone in charge.

CHAPTER EIGHTEEN
THE MAYOR

With Veronica's, Pierre's, and my own constant efforts, we finally managed to secure funding for the film (theoretically at least; the funds were not yet in the bank) from a mix of broadcasters—the ABC, Sundance Channel, TG4 in Ireland, Channel 11 in Thailand, funding agencies, etc. So now I was able to return to Kevin in Kisumu.

Back on track, together with Cathy, we arranged to meet the most important person we could think of in the locality, the mayor of Kisumu.

On a somewhat better-paved road in the middle of the city, there was a boulevard of sorts. We walked up to a concrete building with a big sign saying "Town Hall," which in all these years of filming here I had never before noticed. While women walked busily by, men lounged around the entrance. Kevin nervously passed through, and we walked inside through the open courtyard, up the stairs, to a dark plastic-wood-paneled office where two women were working under flickering fluorescents. One was using a PC that had to be at least ten years old, ancient by modern standards.

Kevin told them, very quietly, that he had an appointment with the mayor. They just looked at him. He repeated himself. They told us to wait for a moment.

Cathy and I went ahead to prepare the mayor for Kevin, leaving him with the two receptionists for the time being. The entrance to her room was through the reception area. We knocked. And a big booming voice told us to "come in."

Priscah Auma Misachi, an imposing woman in her mid-fifties with a huge blue headpiece, rose from behind her wooden desk. She shook our hands and asked where the boy was. We told her he was waiting outside, and that we had wanted to prepare her for the filming. We explained that we were approaching everyone we could, including leaders such as herself, especially as she was the mayor of millions of people in one of the areas worst hit by the epidemic.

We set up our camera and our lights, while she sorted papers on her desk. Finally we called for Kevin, who came shuffling in. (Even when he was nervous, he moved polé polé.)

The mayor rose again from behind her large desk and greeted him, and they sat down to talk.

Kevin told her he was pleased to meet her as a mayor and explained that he was an orphan. She asked if there was no family to help out. He told her there was no family. She looked at me. I nodded that it was true.

She asked how he had managed to go to school, how he had eaten.

He told her about roasting peanuts, how he had snuck into school, how his school fees were now being paid.

She asked him what he wanted to be.

He told her that he wanted to be a doctor.

She nodded, then began to tell him about her life. She said she had wanted to be mayor of Kisumu for twenty-one years. When she was young, she worked hard at school. She got herself into Secretarial College. She passed her exams. She was a secretary for quite a while. Then, in 1984, she decided she wanted to be mayor. She got herself onto the council. Then later she ran for office. She said she lost the first election by one vote, but she kept trying. And finally, last year, she became mayor. So, she said to Kevin, "You can do anything you want if you put your mind to it."

Kevin asked her, as a mayor, what she was doing about AIDS since it was so bad in the community.

She told him that for many years people didn't realize that AIDS was such a big problem; that there had been many superstitions surrounding what it was that was making so many people so sick. But now the government had finally convinced people that it was AIDS. "The awareness has been created. People are aware that HIV and AIDS is a disaster. It's no longer something to joke with. And we are taking a keen care of spreading the gospel of abstaining, to abstain."

Kevin followed up, quietly but determined. "As a mayor, what can you do to counteract the stigmatization? Like the orphans or people not wanting to buy vegetables from people who have HIV." (He was remembering Edwina and her problems, as well as his.)

The mayor looked at him straight on and said, "That is why the government is spending a lot of money in creating awareness. Once you are aware of what causes HIV and AIDS, what makes it infect you, I think people are going to—[and with a big breath here]—abstain."

Kevin asked her this question many different ways. But she repeated the "gospel of abstaining." She also told him again that he could be anything he wanted to be, just like she had wanted to be mayor for twenty-one years. Then we said good-bye and left.

Considering the scientific information Kevin had heard about condoms compared to what he had heard from Albert and now the mayor, Kevin was understandably confused.

I was, too.

CHAPTER NINETEEN

A BRIEF NOTE ABOUT A CONGRESSMAN

The mayor reminded me of a politician I'd once met in the United States a few years earlier, a Republican congressman from the South, a fundamentalist Christian. I had been interviewing him about his faith influencing his politics. At the time, the religious right was advocating abstinence as a major part of sexual education. The movement was also still targeting homosexuality, as it had in the '80s when the epidemic had hit my hometown of New York. I asked the politician then about the AIDS epidemic, and he told me he was proud of voting for the president's package on AIDS, which included funding "abstinence until marriage" as a prevention strategy. "Wasn't that a Christian thing to do," he'd asked, "to give these people in Africa billions of dollars? Even though, even though we understand—"

I had a sense of where he was going with this and tried to interrupt. But he would not be stopped.

"—even though we understand that if they behaved like normal human beings, we wouldn't have this problem."

Just like the mayor of Kisumu—if only they would abstain.

What are normal human beings? Was the young woman Edwina not normal? Jane? Joseph Musyoka? How about many of my friends in heterosexual or gay communities around the world? Or any of the millions of people infected with the HIV virus, the four million more every year? Was it really appropriate to take only certain groups' views of a belief system— such as Christianity—and apply it to a medical "scourge," as the young man in the yellow hat on the streets of Kisumu had called it? (For example, there are well-known religious leaders who are more accepting, such as the courageous Archbishop Desmond Tutu, who in his book *God Has A Dream* welcomes all human love in his understanding of Christianity.)

I felt Kevin deserved better than what the mayor or the congressman were offering. Kevin felt he deserved better than this. We had agreed to seek high and low for answers, so, mindful of Kevin's school schedule, we got permission from his kind schoolteacher, Joy; and Cathy, Kevin, and I decided to go to Nairobi, the nation's capital, where the national leaders were. Perhaps they would have answers worthy of a boy such as Kevin.

Chapter Twenty
The Road to Nairobi

As I've mentioned, before this series of trips to Kenya, I had seen almost nothing of the country. Every time I had been to visit, I would only hang out in the slums of Kisumu or the slums of Mombasa. I hadn't seen anything much beyond these shacks and glimpses of Lake Victoria. More importantly, neither had Kevin.

In Cathy and Jim's Land Rover, we started our trip down to Nairobi. Driving a Land Rover in Africa may seem clichéd, but most clichés exist for a reason. If you want to see the country, these vehicles are great, as the roads in Kenya—even the main highways—are full of holes, and deep ones at that. We piled in, stopped for fuel, and started on our trip. Kevin, as he said, was "not used to being in a car, and the road is very bumpy," so he could only travel for so long before he needed to take a break; but he did very well, looking out the windows at new worlds as they passed.

We stopped briefly at a village that was the childhood home of the former head of Medical Services for the country, Dr. Richard Muga. Here there were many children orphaned by the epidemic.

The village chief, a wiry man in his sixties, and others in the community were taking a novel approach. They wanted to make sure that the children got to keep the small properties of their parents, unlike in other areas where relatives would take the children's inheritance. Here, the orphans were being taught how to grow tea, a crop they could then sell, which could give them a living later on. Otherwise, the chief explained, the children would leave and end up on the streets of the cities.

We met four kids in a field, busily hoeing. They seemed to range from about seven to Kevin's age. An older woman was watching them. Kevin spoke to the children, asking them how they were doing. They said they were fine. They had the same young "adult" look that I had seen when I had first come to Kenya; they acted emotionally self-sufficient. It was the woman who seemed more distraught about their fate. "I'm the one caring for them," she said, "because their mothers died. Their fathers died. Their grandmothers died. Their grandfathers died. So they were alone, so I couldn't leave them."

I don't know what Kevin was thinking as he watched the children. He just stood and watched them. Then it was time to go.

Much of the road to Nairobi is stunningly beautiful. Some of the thatched-roof mud huts and villages along the way over-look lush valleys and mountains. It seems so peaceful. Goats trudge along by the side of the road. And the people walk along the roads as well, slowly, purposefully. I don't want to romanticize what might be real poverty, but there was a part of me that envied the simplicity here, as we passed small dwellings with an acre or two of crops, those goats, and stunning views of the beautiful rolling green hills and valleys. It looked like people were living as they might have thousands of years ago.

Except that, as far as we know, they didn't have this epidemic then.

Kevin hadn't been this far before, and he continued to stare out the window intently. His parents had come from villages like these, as had his other relatives who'd passed away.

A few years earlier, I'd been in a similar region in Malawi, in a place called Nkhota Nkhota, right by the stunning and huge Lake Malawi, facing Tanzania. This was not far from where Stanley found his hero Livingstone with those famous words, "Dr. Livingstone, I presume." Except now the country was in the midst of a famine.

We had been filming with representatives of a major international nongovernmental organization, who were showing us their program of home-based care where the villagers would tend to each other. However, these villages that the NGO was developing its models on were right by the road. Here, where the charity could more easily deliver aid, it was hard to really see the effects of famine, the hunger-stricken look we've all become used to seeing on the news.

Up in Nkhota Nkhota, the owner of the lodge we were

staying at, an Englishman named John, was definitely at odds with the NGO people even though they had recommended his place. He said that, if we wanted to see the effect of HIV/AIDS and the famine, we should go inland. We should walk off the road to where the majority of the Malawians lived, not where the shiny white UN-style vehicles found it easier to go.

We had one day left for filming. So we'd set off, Christian, John, and I. We walked as far off-road as we could get in the hours we still had left.

Here, we repeatedly came across small groups of round huts, basically empty but for some old women and children. The corn that did grow was in tiny patches, sad and brown. We talked to an old woman, tired, wrinkled, her grandchildren hovering about her. The men had died. Her daughters had died, leaving her behind with these children. She sat forlornly on the stone porch of her hut. When we finished talking, the children still stayed by her side. They were not emaciated, like Joseph Musyoka had been, but they were thin, too thin. And their eyes were too sorrowful, as they clutched her own thin flesh.

I remembered that grandmother now in Kenya as we drove down past fieldworkers with their children in the lush green tea fields of Kericho, then through the Rift Valley as we headed steadily toward Nairobi, past signs declaring "Happy Churches," churches of every stripe and color, and every once in a while signs for Voluntary Testing and Counseling Centers for HIV/AIDS.

We took Kevin to Lake Nkuru, a virtual city of pink flamingoes in the beautifully still water, all murmuring, chatting quietly. He looked out over the lake in wonder. He had never seen anything like this. This was where the tourists, like myself, would come to see the zebras, the gazelles, the extraordinary beauty of the landscape of Kenya, of Africa.

We kept going. We needed to get to Nairobi before dark. Carjackings were rampant in the city, especially at night.

We passed more signs promising big gospel events and Jesus's love.

As night fell, we kept driving, occasional headlights passing us on the road, listening to the radio. Hours later, exhausted, with the passing headlights now more frequent, we made it to Nairobi and the guarded gate of Cathy's apartment. (Many houses are guarded due to the high rate of robbery and murder.)

Cathy showed Kevin to his room. Kevin looked around it, finding a place to neatly put the few clothes he had brought in his knapsack. We all had a quick dinner, and then it was time for bed. Kevin went to his room and eventually turned his light off—in this room with electricity!

CHAPTER TWENTY-ONE
WHAT ORPHANS LEARN IN NAIROBI

In the morning, Kevin just stood at the door of the bathroom, bemused by all the unfamiliar plumbing, staring at the shower.

Where Kevin lived, there were only public showers, which cost ten shillings. For the same amount of money, he could get plenty of water from the neighbors to clean himself with over a week. It was no reflection on Kevin that he couldn't afford a shower. Instead, it was to his credit that he kept himself and his shirts so clean considering his circumstances.

Cathy showed him how to take a shower, explaining how to turn on the tap and how to get a good balance between hot and cold water. Once he understood, he waited fully clothed for us to leave. He grew to like showers a great deal.

In Nairobi, Kevin was also very worried that his clothes would be dirty for when he'd have to go back to school, that he wouldn't have time to wash them. As I made him toast and

Cathy made coffee, he continued to fret about it. I was starting to discover that Kevin was a worrier. Once a worry took hold of him, it wouldn't let go. So I took his clothes next door to Cathy's friend Singa's apartment. And, as Kevin watched, quietly and a bit incredulously, I put them in the washing machine. He watched as I shut the door and the machine began its cycle, turning the clothes around and around in the sudsy water. (But I don't think it could do a better job than Kevin.)

In the daylight, we explored downtown Nairobi, a place you don't walk around at night, whether muzungu or African.

A twentieth-century creation, the city of Nairobi is a mass of '60s and '70s high-rises, with a massive amount of traffic on the road and masses of people on the street. Some large buses come and go filled to the brim with passengers, but the main public transport system consists of brightly colored matatus, privately owned vans, with vivid decals like "Whom God bless, let no one curse" and pictures of Bob Marley or Michael Jordan, which stop at a moment's notice in the midst of traffic while the "conductor," usually a young man, quickly ushers people in.

One place of charm is the old train station, where beautiful old brown trains operate on a line created over a hundred years ago by the British colonialists with unfortunately few improvements since.

To Kevin, compared to Kisumu, downtown Nairobi was a mind-boggling hustle and bustle. He had visited the capital once before, many years ago, but only for a few hours. He had gone from the airport into the city and back, in the company of Father Hans, the founder of Pandipieri Catholic Centre.

Walking around this dense place was another thing entirely. As Kevin said, "One can get quite lost."

There was one point quite late in the day when I found myself worrying that this might have happened.

Kevin was supposed to be waiting with Cathy and a driver we had for the day, while I went off to check e-mails (and see if any money had finally gone into the bank). Kevin told Cathy he was just going to go to the corner. When I got back, Cathy and the driver were in the car. She told me Kevin had said he was just going to stand by the corner. I went to the corner. No Kevin to be found.

I looked up and down the block and couldn't see him. I started panicking, walking up the blocks this way and that. We had taken this boy's life in our hands and brought him to the city in which, as he said, one could get lost, and now it seemed he had. It was witching hour and not safe, particularly for a boy from Kisumu. I raced to and fro, heart pounding, until finally, fifteen minutes later, Kevin came sauntering back in that polé polé Kenyan way. I asked him where he'd gone. He didn't know. He'd just "kind of wandered off." I told him I'd been terribly worried. He admitted he'd been a bit scared himself; the streets were much more confusing than in Kisumu. I made him promise not to wander off again, unless he got my permission. I felt like I was talking to a toddler, not a seventeen-year-old!

Kevin wanted to meet other young people impacted by the epidemic, so we were going to visit two friends of mine here who were also orphans: Ann Njeri and Evelyn Shiro (our nurse and jet pilot). They were now in Nairobi attending a Seventh

Day Adventist school, having been sent there by Lucy Yinda and her Wema Centre in Mombasa.

Both Ann and Evelyn had been street children until the age of about twelve. I'd got to know them when making *14 Million Dreams.* Ann had told me honestly about having to have "a sugar daddy" (a man you have sex with for money) by the age of eleven. Evelyn had been addicted to sniffing glue. Lucy took them in, welcoming Ann after she was arrested, with Evelyn coming later. Now Lucy was "Mum." Wema Centre housed about two hundred girls, and ensured they all went to primary school. If they qualified for secondary education, Lucy found the money from somewhere.

Back when we'd filmed *14 Million Dreams,* Christian and I had worked with Ann and Evelyn—with Lucy as chaperone—and re-created their lives on the street. Lucy had suggested we go near one of the nightclubs where girls just a few years older would be with their "sugar daddies." When we'd tried to film, one drunken patron came out and started yelling at us. "I am a native person," he screamed. He set off a literal riot on the streets as more drunken "persons" and patrons came after us. Lucy; the dedicated Timothy Kinyoda, who worked with her helping street children; the girls; and Christian and I all immediately ran into the club for protection. It was a growing madhouse outside. In the club, girls just a year or two older than Evelyn and Ann stared at us angrily—we were making their patrons uncomfortable. The proprietor asked us to leave. Into the mob?

Then the police came! It turned out that while we were

hiding in the club, someone had smashed the windows of the Wells Fargo building next door and set off the alarms. An armed militia had shown up, bringing on the police, who insisted on taking Timothy into the station for questioning. Christian and I told him he didn't need to go, but he went with them, saying it would all be fine. Lucy tried to call her contacts in the judiciary on her mobile phone, but none of them could be found.

Our driver eventually braved the madness (as no one out there even knew who he was) and made it to our truck. He called us just as he pulled up outside the club and we ran out to him, jumping in as he sped off, tires screeching.

We went to the police station demanding to see Timothy. The officer on duty swore he had no idea what we were talking about and that no one had been arrested, not in the last few hours. In a very Inspector Clouseau moment, as the officer continued to swear there was no one there, Timothy walked out from behind him accompanied by another guard! He was free to go.

The drunk who'd started the riot was also there. He asked us for a lift back to the club. We told him to walk!

The next day we thought the girls needed a positive experience after that whole debacle, which we could now fortunately laugh about. So Lucy brought Ann and Evelyn and the other girls from Wema over to her brother's hotel (where we were staying), and we all watched the World Cup on television in the main room, Ireland against Spain. The German tourists wondered at the girls, who immediately got into the game. Ann and

Evelyn rooted for Ireland, the underdogs in the match—who came very close to winning.

Now both girls were as far from the streets of Mombasa as one could be. They were staying at the Seventh Day Adventist campus, a boarding school for boys and girls. We went there to meet them. Kevin stood on the huge soccer field looking out enviously at all the kids in uniform playing, while I went to find Ann and Evelyn.

When Ann came down to meet him, Kevin grew very shy, but Ann's forthrightness soon brought him right out of it. She then brought him over to Evelyn and explained that Kevin was an orphan, like them, but that he lived alone. Evelyn was shocked to hear that.

The three sat down on the grass comparing their lives. Ann and Evelyn told him about life on the street, which Kevin seemed horrified by. Evelyn had originally lived on the streets of Nairobi. But after the bombing of the U.S. embassy, she said, the streets had become too dangerous. She and some friends had then made their way down to Mombasa. They told Kevin about Lucy; that she was like their mother now.

There was a hint of longing on his face, as he listened to them tell how they felt safe at Wema. They felt cared for. They loved Lucy. And Lucy loved them. And here at this school, they also felt safe. Kevin asked them what they did on school holidays. On short ones, they stayed with Lucy's mother here in Nairobi. On longer ones, they went back to Mombasa. Their scholarships were being paid for by the Danish government.

They were both incredulous that Kevin lived by himself.

Wasn't he scared? Didn't he have nightmares? What did he do on school holidays? At Christmas?

Kevin told them that yes, sometimes it was scary. And when he was younger, it had been very scary. Now he felt better, but it was still lonely.

Watching this, I felt even worse than I had already about that decision we adults had all made to leave him in the community.

Ann began to act more shyly (and coy) with Kevin than I'd normally seen her. Her eyes were sometimes cast down, long lashes fluttering as she asked him questions.

They then talked about what they were learning in school, before moving on to what they were being taught about AIDS. Evelyn told Kevin that their biology teacher, Simon Koicho, had told them to abstain. Not to use condoms. He'd told them that condoms had microscopic holes that the virus could get through. I very much wanted to hear this teacher talking to a class, so I went to organize that.

Finally, we said our good-byes to the girls, but only after promising that we would come back and take them to eat at the Village Market nearby at some point. At the Seventh Day Adventist school the girls were only allowed to eat vegetarian food. Village Market was basically a Western-style shopping mall and included lots of different eateries in an open-air food court. More importantly, those eateries served meat! Ann and Evelyn were desperate for some chicken.

I promised.

CHAPTER TWENTY-TWO
CHICKEN AND FRENCH FRIES, AND DARTH VADER

Chicken was also Kevin's favorite food. I realized I hadn't been paying enough attention to his diet. When we were in Kisumu and would eat out somewhere, Kevin would always order chicken, primarily chicken and French fries. Now that we were in Nairobi, we needed to eat out quite often. Kevin would immediately want chicken and French fries.

I asked him if he had learned about nutrition. He gave me a blank look. Then I told him that there was absolutely no value in eating French fries and, if he wanted to do well in school, he needed to eat better.

This was a fact. He could get very absentminded, and he'd told me his grades were falling off. But having raised himself, how much could he be expected to know about nutrition? Most of the people where he lived survived on a staple of ugali, which is basically white cornmeal, almost a pure carbohydrate with no vitamins or nutrients. But it was cheap and stuffed your belly. The next time we went to get something to eat, I asked him what he wanted.

"You tell me what to eat, Miles," he replied. "You choose for me."

"Do you want chicken and salad? Or maybe some nice beef?"

"You choose. You know what is good for me."

Instead of the typical teenager normally demanding more autonomy and freedom, Kevin, who'd had too much autonomy and freedom, wanted me to tell him what to do! That was Kevin's form of rebellion. And that's how I became Kevin's nutritionist in Nairobi, and even back in Kisumu when we returned there with him. Even when we would leave him to have dinner alone back in his shack, I'd first go to a restaurant and choose something healthy for him to eat: fish, with salad and vegetables. If chicken, then chicken with vegetables.

I worried that someone his age coming from a slum and accustomed to a very limited and impoverished diet would find it difficult trying different kinds of foods. In Nairobi, however, Kevin became something of a gourmand as he hung out with Cathy; her husband, Jim; Singa; and myself after we had finished filming and discussing AIDS for the day.

To thank Jim and Cathy for their hospitality in putting Kevin up and Singa for putting me up, I wanted to take us all to dinner. It could be argued that exposing Kevin to "fine dining" when he came from the slums of Kisumu was unfair. But I'd grown up on the poor side, yet was treated to some extraordinary meals by rich friends of my parents, and my parents had also splurged on special occasions. I felt Kevin deserved to be exposed to the best we could afford, now that we were in Nairobi. And some money had also finally cleared in the bank account!

Cathy and Jim suggested Japanese for this dinner, mentioning that here in Nairobi there was a lovely Japanese restaurant. I was doubtful and nervous about the idea, that it might be just too different for Kevin, but he seemed keen. Which was odd. Most Kenyans I have met like *nyama choma,* a form of grilled meat, or they like their chicken. But everything is prepared with almost no salt and certainly no spice.

Once, when a Kenyan crew and I were filming at an Indian temple, and were fed Indian dishes, the crew could not stand the spicy food. They could barely make it through the ice cream. I also remember sharing a flight with a Kenyan official who told me how much he'd liked living in America for the six months he was there, except for one thing. The food was awful; too spicy, too salty.

Yet . . . I have a lovely photograph of Kevin learning how to eat with chopsticks at the Japanese restaurant. As a proud Kenyan chef, trained by the Japanese to be an excellent sushi chef, served our table, Kevin gamely tried everything. He tried spicy tuna roll. He tried hot wasabi mustard—and liked it, laughing at how hot it was. He ate sashimi (raw fish), too. Beyond the pleasure of watching him enjoy himself so much messing around with the chopsticks, I was proud of him. As his nutritionist.

On varying days and on subsequent trips, Kevin tried different foods, ranging from Thai to Italian. Some of it was cooked at Cathy's house, as Jim was an excellent cook and enjoyed preparing meals for us. The dish Kevin liked best was a passion that both he and Jim shared: roast chicken. That was something special for Sunday night. (It was not served with French fries but vegetables!)

I also realized I had to watch how I spoke, as did Cathy. We had a tendency to swear when shots we were trying to get didn't go quite our way, or there was too much traffic, etc.—like many other adults. But we didn't have an adult with us. We had an impressionable young man. So we tried to limit the use of words such as "dammit" or "f—king." I certainly know now that we were not always successful in this, but we tried.

On another night, I promised Kevin we'd go to the movies, which he was very excited about. The only films he'd ever seen were some Nigerian videos that were played at a shack nearby, where mainly young men came to watch for about ten shillings a view.

On movie night, Kevin and I went with Singa to the cinema at the Village Market. We rushed through the mall-like space to try and get to the theater on time. The new, and final, Star Wars movie was showing and that seemed like something Kevin would enjoy, but we were running late. There'd be no time for dinner. I treated us all to the tickets, and Singa bought Kevin popcorn, soda, and some lollies while Singa and I had hot dogs. (The "nutritionist" had to stay silent.)

We sat down in the big screening room; there were not that many people in the cinema, even though it was a Saturday night. Perhaps it was not too popular; perhaps few could afford the tickets beyond the middle class.

The movie began.

Watching Kevin watch the movie on the big screen with the "Stereo Sound" was more entertaining than watching the movie itself. He was absolutely engrossed, transfixed, transported into the life of the young Darth Vader.

We stayed through every last credit, Kevin watching even these. When the lights came up, Kevin turned to us, his eyes wide with amazement and with the broadest smile on his face. "That was wonderful," he said. "It was wonderful."

For the rest of the evening he seemed to be replaying the movie in his head.

And then there was the movie we were making together, where he was the hero, endlessly getting into the Land Rover spaceship and going from leader to leader to see if we could stop the evil from spreading.

But who was Darth Vader in our story? "The enemy is the virus," said Sean Emery. "The enemy is the virus."

CHAPTER TWENTY-THREE
CONSPIRACIES AND ABSTINENCE

We returned to Ann and Evelyn's school to see their biology teacher conduct a class about condoms and whether they could stop the enemy. We found Ann Njeri and Evelyn, and they found Simon Koicho, the teacher, for us. Simon then brought us along to his class. Kevin sat next to Ann. The other students were all the same age, late teens, hormones raging.

Simon wore a white lab coat. He spoke very clearly, passionately, and did seem, as he had told us, to have a good grasp of biology. There were other things that were questionable. He started by explaining that the only way one could avoid AIDS was by "abstaining from what?" he asked, pausing for dramatic effect. "Sex!" Condoms did work with some STDs, he admitted. But they did not work with HIV/AIDS. Contrary to the scientific evidence we'd heard, he said there were very small holes through which the virus could travel. He explained the difference between HIV and AIDS. That HIV is the virus itself, and that AIDS is the syndrome. He drew diagrams on the board, explaining how HIV replicates itself.

He then explained a theory that other Africans I've met believe: that HIV was invented in the United States. However, his theory of why and how I hadn't heard before. According to Simon, it was invented by the U.S. military to kill off the African Americans when they got the vote. The military feared that if the African American population kept growing, it might outvote the white population. (Considering the stories Africans have heard of the medical experiments done on African American men in the 1930s to see what would happen if they were not treated for syphilis; and of the black soldiers, the Tuskegee Airmen in World War II, who were injected with syphilis, this is not perhaps as irrational a theory as it might first appear.)

But, Simon continued, the military had invented something that could no longer be contained only in the black population. Gay white men had contracted the virus and had then got AIDS as well. He quoted from the American writer Randy Shilts's book *And the Band Played On*. Shilts had begun writing about what was then called GRID (gay-related immunodeficiency diseases) in 1982, and documented how the gay community was, as he said, "virtually engineered to ensure the rapid proliferation of a sexually transmitted disease. And people did not really do anything about it." Shilts had documented how public health officials did not take the epidemic seriously in America.

Now, said Simon, the AIDS epidemic no longer killed just

the African Americans but everyone. This was the reason the United States had let out the secret of HIV/AIDS to the world. Now they needed a worldwide response to try to control the epidemic.

Kevin and Ann Njeri exchanged flirtatious looks a few times, as Simon, in front of all these seventeen-year-olds with normal seventeen-year-old hormones raging, continued.

Simon did like President Bush, because of his pro-Christian stance. "The reason why President Bush is saying that we should abstain is that Bush is not out to kill black Americans now. And even the Africans. They have discovered the virus is destroying every human being." And the only solution was what?

"Abstinence."

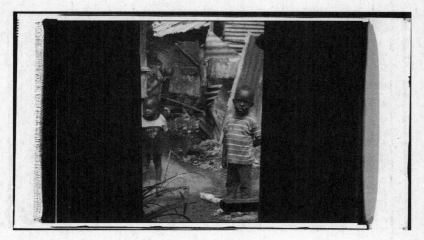

ABOVE: Two of Kevin's neighbours outside his home.

BELOW: Maxwell and Sennye on campus in Melbourne.

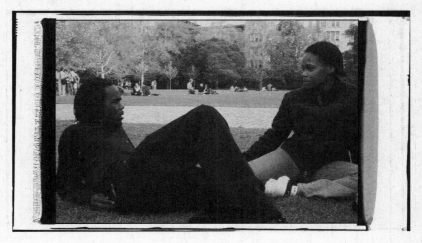

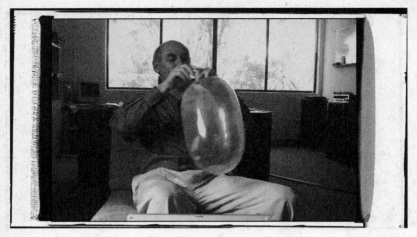

ABOVE: John Gerofi of Enersol in Sydney tying up a balloon, just made from a condom!

BELOW: Kevin walks along the shores of beautiful Lake Nkuru, past a city of flamingoes.

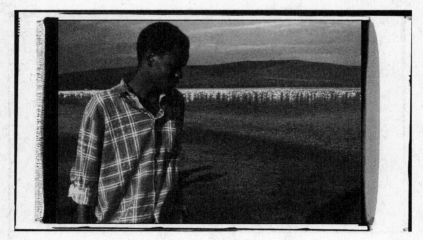

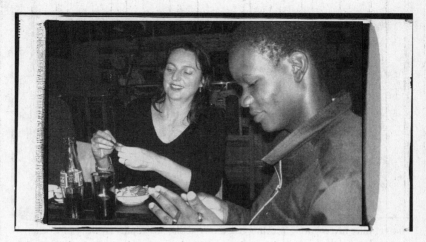

ABOVE: Cathy Scott teaching Kevin how to use chopsticks at a Japanese restaurant in Nairobi.

BELOW: Kevin and Humphrey at the graveyard for children who died of HIV/AIDS at Nyumbani.

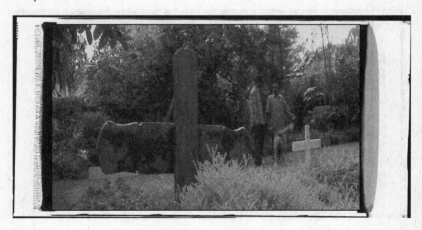

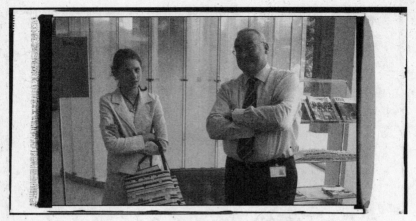

ABOVE: Julia investigating 'Kevin's Questions' with Christopher Murray of Roche, the pharmaceutical company.

BELOW: A Kenyan open-air market.

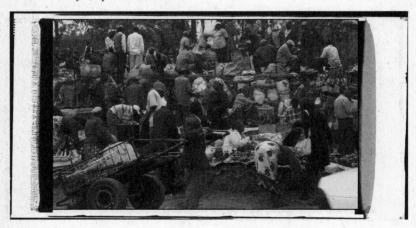

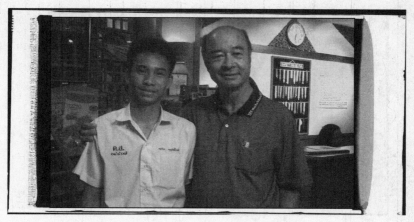

ABOVE: Ponlapat after his interview with Senator Mechai Viravaidya, at his restaurant Cabbages and Condoms in Bangkok, Thailand.

BELOW: Street boys of Nairobi. One of these children told me how much he wanted to go to school.

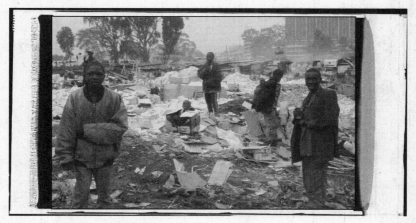

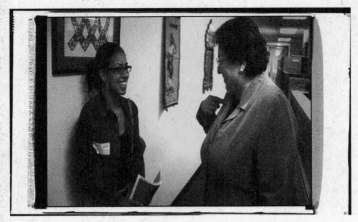

ABOVE: Carolina with Thoraya Obaid, executive director of UNFPA, talking about the teenager's prom dress.

BELOW: Outside his home, as neighbours look on, Kevin reads the book Jeffrey Sachs autographed for him.

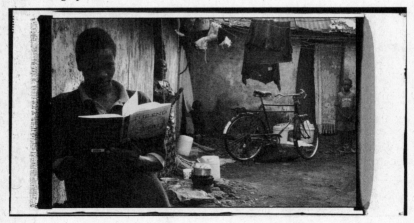

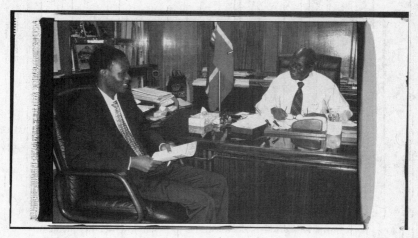

ABOVE: Kevin (in his new suit) meets Dr Moody Awori, the vice president of Kenya.

BELOW: Evelyn, Cathy, Ann, me and Kevin after the chicken feast at Village Market.

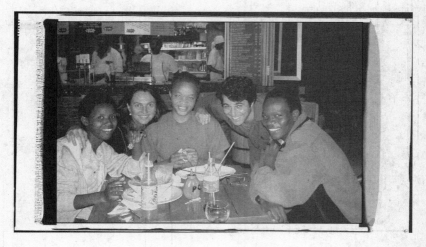

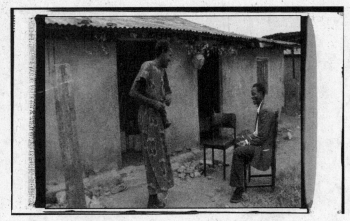

ABOVE: Jane, formerly bedridden, demonstrates to Kevin how well her medicine works — by dancing!

BELOW: Kevin looks with earned pride at the pictures of himself and the vice president of his country.

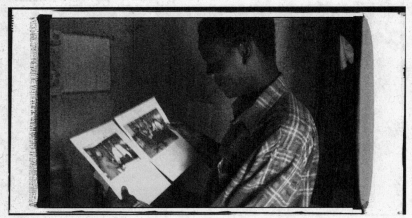

Chapter Twenty-four
Meeting the Archbishop

In the center of town, right near the Intercontinental Hotel, where many "intercontinental" conferences are held, is a large Catholic church, the church that Ndingi Mwana a'Nzeki, the archbishop of Nairobi, presides over.

The church was packed. Kevin sat, listening to early afternoon Mass. His face was quiet and attentive, one in a sea of devoted faces, mainly men and women in their twenties and upwards. They were black; the Jesus on the cross was white. The archbishop, a well-kept man in his seventies, was giving a sermon about family values.

When it came time to take communion, Kevin didn't get up and join the queue. I wondered if that was in protest, but he later told me it was because he had not been confirmed. Of course. How would he have had time to prepare for that?

A few days later, very early on a Sunday morning, we drove up to the archbishop's residence. Kevin got out at the security gate and pushed the buzzer, saying it was "Kevin to see the archbishop." The electric gate swung open.

We waited in a dark reception area, with pictures of the archbishop's predecessors on the walls. Some were white. Some were black. Kevin looked up at them quietly. He didn't want to take a wrong turn here. Cathy and I probably were a bit too jokey, commenting on all the pictures of the various archbishops on the walls. Perhaps we were nervous for him—but Kevin didn't respond to us. He stood in the room looking at all the imagery. Cathy and I politely shut up.

Finally, dressed in his robes, the archbishop came in. "Where do you want to do this?" he asked matter-of-factly.

We sat on the porch, Kevin facing him. At first the archbishop was somewhat hostile, especially toward Cathy and me. He said he didn't want to be misrepresented by the press. He felt the press always twisted his words, and he was not amused. I promised to represent what he said fairly and not take him out of context. He still didn't lighten up.

But as Kevin listened to him quietly, intently, and then told him about his priest at St Joseph's church in Kisumu, the man grew warmer and answered Kevin's questions gently. By the end, as he heard Kevin's story about being an orphan, he was actually kindly.

"How do you prevent AIDS?" Kevin asked.

The archbishop answered straightforwardly. "To married people, be faithful to one another. Unmarried people, the Catholic Church supports abstention, to abstain from sex. The Catholic Church does not accept condoms. The use of it for the Catholic Church is out, and we are very adamant. To approve condoms is to approve something that will bring a very bad effect on our people."

When Kevin asked him about the efficacy of condoms, he said young people had them in their pockets and still they got AIDS. They got drunk, and so they didn't use them.

He did tell Kevin that it was all right for married people, if one of them was HIV positive, to use condoms. This was, for him, a radical departure from his earlier days of completely banning them. (Although his approach was more liberal than the papal line, which forbid condoms, period, as of 2005.)

The archbishop told Kevin, "AIDS is not God's punishment. It is not. God is a God of mercy. It is we who enter into these situations. See, people can abstain. People do abstain. But even Jesus said, 'We are all sinners. Let he who is without sin cast the first stone.'"

Kevin asked him, "What does the Catholic Church do to [sic] orphans?"

The archbishop told him about Nyumbani, an orphanage for HIV-positive children whom no one else in Kenya would take, children who were stigmatized.

The archbishop was very proud of Nyumbani as a Catholic institution.

When they had finished the interview, the archbishop and Kevin walked in the garden, the older man encouraging Kevin to study hard.

Oddly enough, Nyumbani would be the turning point for Kevin, and his initiation into the complexities of faith, the HIV/AIDS issue, and abstinence and condoms.

CHAPTER TWENTY-FIVE
NYUMBANI AND HUMPHREY

Cathy had told me about Nyumbani as well. My initial reaction to it had been skeptical. A Catholic orphanage run by an American priest, Father Angelo D'Agostino, just smelled like bad news to me. I had seen some religious orphanages in Mombasa, albeit run by evangelical groups, where kids had to sing hymns on a daily basis for their daily bread, and I'd also heard some people question some of the methods of D'Agostino. However, he was well regarded by many, and he did get through to the government, even getting the president's wife, the first lady of Kenya, to visit and support his orphanages. Cathy had been very impressed when she'd met him, and now that we'd heard how proud of Nyumbani the archbishop was, it was obviously something we had to check out.

When we first drove in, my heart sank. The compound was nice enough looking—plain stone buildings, with a raised

"African" hut, a sandbox and playground in the center—but I could hear kids singing hymns. At the far end of the compound was a white building, a converted schoolroom, in which Father D'Agostino was holding Mass. He was a short, rather stout white man with a goatee, wearing a tie-dye robe in swirling purples and oranges, very '60s. He was officiating with a black priest, Father Protus Lumiti, dressed more traditionally in a suit with the collar. Young children all sat in the front, some on benches, some on chairs. In the middle and the back were the older kids, some white guests, a few nuns, and some of the other workers, I guessed. Kevin went to sit in the back and just watched.

As Mass continued, I went outside. Some white kids from a religious college in Texas were there visiting and wanted to know what we were doing. My heart continued sinking. I watched Kevin engage in the part of Catholic ceremonies I like, the community part, when neighbor turns to neighbor and says, "Peace be with you." "And with you."

When it came time for communion, while all the children even younger than him went up to Father D'Agostino, Kevin stayed behind. And I felt more of a pang than I had at the big Nairobi church. Even this—simple communion—something Kevin would have liked, he was denied. Even the children at the orphanage here had access to this if they wanted.

Afterward, we met Father D'Agostino in the midst of all the people keen to see him, and Father Protus Lumiti, who managed the orphanage.

More importantly, we wanted to meet the kids at the orphanage. How did they like it here? Honestly.

After speaking briefly, D'Agostino left us to talk with the kids, as he had many things to do—and all those visitors to attend to, white visitors like me.

A beautiful thing about filming young people is that they constantly trip you up. And in the best way possible. For the film, we wanted to find one person to get to know, someone whom Kevin could relate to. And so we began to cast who this would be.

A group of teenagers came over at this point and, as Kevin seemed too shy to speak to them, Cathy and I took over. As we talked to each of the kids, asking them how they'd arrived at the orphanage and how they liked the school, Kevin just watched.

As Cathy and I started to discuss who we thought would be most appropriate to film talking to Kevin, we turned to get his opinion. But while we were yakking, he'd already made his choice and was walking off with Humphrey, a boy one year younger than him in a bright purple shirt. They were already deep in conversation, so we hurried to catch up with them.

Kevin and Humphrey walked, followed by a lovely old golden retriever, as the boy told Kevin about his life. HIV positive and an orphan, Humphrey had first lived somewhere else that he could not remember and then came here. Just as Ann and Evelyn loved Lucy, so he loved and admired Father D'Agostino. When the orphanage had moved to Nyumbani, the government primary school in the district would not let the HIV-positive children attend, and D'Agostino and Lumiti had to pay fees for private schooling. The students in the public school were afraid of such children, and the government (at that point, under the dictatorship of Daniel Arap Moi) was no help. So Father D'Agostino and Father Lumiti sued the government to force the school to allow the orphans in. They won—in early 2004.

But, Humphrey told Kevin, it still wasn't easy. When they first got to the school, all the other children shunned them. "When the other pupils discovered we were from Nyumbani, they were shocked. They wouldn't be close to us. There was nothing we could do about it."

He continued telling Kevin that the other kids in the class sat on the other side of the room, scared by the myths they might have heard from their parents—that they would get the disease by talking to the orphans, or even by eating with them. It was easy to tell which children were from the orphanage, because their clothes had the word "Nyumbani" on them.

Of course, though, since people would not admit to having AIDS, who knew how many of these children's parents were HIV positive, or in fact if they themselves were infected? (In fact, Nyumbani ran a testing center for the community!)

After a while, Humphrey and some of the other kids from the orphanage tore the name off their clothes to see if that could make them fit in better, but they were already marked. However, gradually, the other kids began to talk to them. They didn't all become best friends, but at least they talked, and were accepted finally.

Kevin and Humphrey continued walking and talking, with the golden retriever tagging along, right in between them, happily wagging its tail. As Cathy and I took a break, Kevin went off to sit and have lunch in one of the little houses around the square with Humphrey and the other kids: some rice, what looked like *githeri*—a corn-and-bean dish—and chicken. Kevin sat down with them, talked with them all, ate with them all. Cathy and I found them and filmed them as a group, laughing and chatting; some of the littler boys vied for each other's food, looking at the others' bowls, even though there was plenty for seconds on the stove. The scene reminded me of my brother, sister, and me at the dinner table, each knowing the other's food was better!

Afterward, Kevin told me he was glad we filmed them eating: he wanted to show other people that it was okay to eat with HIV-positive children.

Later, in Humphrey's shared room, Humphrey sat on the top bunk of the bed, and Kevin stood, leaning against the wooden railing, and they talked more about HIV. Mindful of what he'd heard from everyone from Albert to the archbishop, Kevin asked Humphrey, a Catholic like himself, what he'd been taught at the orphanage "so as not to transmit it."

Humphrey told Kevin that first, as Humphrey was HIV positive, if he got a cut and Kevin got a cut, you shouldn't mix blood. Kevin nodded. He understood that. Then Humphrey turned Kevin's mind around. He told Kevin that the Father had told them that when they grew up, abstinence was a 100 percent sure way of preventing the transmission of HIV, and condoms were 99 percent sure. But the Father had said, "If you can't abstain and be 100 percent sure, it's better to be 99 percent sure."

Kevin was shocked to hear this from Humphrey, that his priest would say this. Having heard so much talk about "abstinence only" for so long, so was I.

Humphrey repeated what he said, nodding: yes, this is what he'd been taught. "If you can't be 100 percent sure, it's better to be 99 percent sure."

Later, outside, we found D'Agostino, now dressed in a more conservative gray sweater. Kevin asked him about condoms and said that, as a Catholic, he had been taught not to use condoms—period. So, how could D'Agostino, a Catholic priest, tell his orphans they could use condoms?

D'Agostino then explained how he thought, still from a very Catholic perspective but contrary to the archbishop—and even the Pope himself in 2005—that one could use condoms. "The Catholic Church has a policy that seems to be against the use of condoms. But the basic moral theology of the Catholic Church has two principles which would allow the use of condoms. One is the principle of the unjust aggressor. If a person is about to kill you, you are allowed to defend yourself and kill that person. Likewise, in the case of AIDS, using a condom to prevent the transmission of a fatal disease is permissible. Another one is the principle of double effect. If you do something with a good intention, but it has another side effect that is not so good, you're not responsible for the side effect. You're only responsible for the good effect. So using a condom, you're trying to prevent the transmission of a disease, not prevent procreation."

Kevin's mind reeled.

And my last aversion to Nyumbani disappeared.

CHAPTER TWENTY-SIX

MEDICINE AND ORPHANS

When Sarah and I were in Amsterdam, as she was attending the institute most of the time, I had my days free to work on my own projects. Some of the day I would spend shopping in the street markets. We stayed near the Tropen Museum, a museum primarily devoted to the Netherlands' relationship with its former colonies. The area is predominantly Muslim, with fantastic shops and stalls run by people from North Africa, Suriname, and, of course, the Netherlands. Often, I would bicycle around just sightseeing.

I took off one day late in November 2004, after I'd returned from my first reunion with Kevin. I rode away from the center of town, farther and farther away, past the park my wife loved with its friendly rooster and chickens. Far away from the city center, I found another park. I locked up the bicycle and went for a wander. In it, I discovered a small cemetery, with perhaps a thousand or so graves. It was a children's cemetery.

A few parents stood by some of the graves. On several, pictures of the children had been placed. Nearly every grave had toys and sweets on it. Some had teddy bears. There were small Christmas trees with gifts underneath them. It was around St. Nicholas Day, when presents are given in the Netherlands.

St. Nicholas I remembered from my own youth, as I went to a school with a Germanic background, the Rudolf Steiner school. Nicholas looked an awful lot like Santa Claus, only he had a helper named Ruprecht, who wore blackface (now very controversial in the Netherlands).

The cemetery was heartbreaking. So many lives, ended so quickly. So much grief. So much love from the parents, still giving their precious children gifts—literally for the afterlife. "After life."

Six months later at Nyumbani, Kevin and Humphrey walked past the schoolhouse that also served as the church, through a garden to the small cemetery at the orphanage. There were little white crosses with names on them, maybe fifteen in all. These were not all the children that had died at Nyumbani, but all the children who had no relatives to claim them. These are some of the names and dates:

Dennis Misati, 4/5/93–2/1/2000
Carmela Kwok, 10/28/95–1/1/96
Rose Gacheri, 9/1/99–5/10/2000
Joan Zawadi, 11/19/90–12/26/96 . . .
one day after Christmas.

There were no Christmas gifts or gifts from St. Nicholas on these graves. There were no parents to leave presents for these children.

Kevin and Humphrey stood at the graves quietly. The old golden retriever followed and waited with the boys. Humphrey told Kevin, "A long time ago, we didn't have medicines, so these people here, they died, because we didn't have medicine."

For a long time, the orphanage was unable to get any antiretrovirals for the children. The drugs were very expensive and hard to come by, and the Kenyan government wouldn't break international patent laws and buy generics.

Brazil and India were two countries that had broken with the Western pharmaceutical giants' patents monopoly. By manufacturing generics themselves, Brazil at that time, in 2001, was providing HIV drugs to 90,000 people, when Africa—where the majority of AIDS patients were—had no generic drugs. The cost of the treatment for a year provided by either the Indian or Brazilian companies at the time was $350, as opposed to the $10,000 it would cost to treat a patient in the United States.

The Kenyan government, however, was wedded to foreign aid. It claimed it was not in a position to break the patent laws. So bringing in these generic drugs was a crime. When D'Agostino had first tried to get medicines in for his orphans, he was blocked by the government. So the orphanage could not access the antiretroviral drug therapies that might keep the children at Nyumbani alive. However, D'Agostino, a medical doctor by training, was determined to save his kids, regardless of the Kenyan government. With the high profile that Nyumbani had, when pressed, Kenyan officials let it be known that they would not arrest Father D'Agostino. The orphanage became the first place in Africa to import generic drugs, donated by a Brazilian company.

As Kevin looked over the graves, Humphrey continued. "Now Father brought us the medicines here to Nyumbani, and there are some people who have survived here and some people died. And me myself," Humphrey said proudly, thumping his chest, "I survived." Humphrey told Kevin that he was now on the antiretrovirals (ARVs). He took pills every day, administered by the nurse at the orphanage. These pills were keeping him, and all the other children like him at the orphanage, alive. There are about one hundred children at the orphanage of Nyumbani. Before the drugs, two or three children used to die every month. No child has died since 2002.

Kevin asked Humphrey how many of these people in these graves were Humphrey's friends.

"Three of them: James Ali, Samson, and Felix."

Kevin then asked a very simple question.

"Was any of them your best friend?"

(I remembered when I had "best friends" in elementary or high school. Sometimes we had fights and stopped being best friends. But not because one or the other of us died.)

Was any of them your best friend?

Humphrey pointed to a grave in the corner. "James Ali there, he was my best friend ever."

Humphrey went and sat by the grave of his friend James Ali.

James Ali, 12/15/91-7/22/02 RIP

As Humphrey sat, his arms around his legs, head on his chin, the old golden retriever came and put his paw on Humphrey's arm. Humphrey kept staring at the gravesite of his friend. The dog insisted. It would not be ignored, and put its paw on Humphrey again. Humphrey couldn't help but give the smallest smile.

The question—"Does it matter to anyone if there is one less of us?"—seems pertinent here.

It mattered very much to Humphrey that his best friend was not here. But I was glad the old golden retriever still was.

Another project Nyumbani runs is the Lea Toto program, established to support HIV-positive children living with their families or other caretakers in the surrounding areas and in Nairobi. Nyumbani has its own laboratory for HIV testing, to monitor the children and service the community. (Allegations were made against Nyumbani, including some by Dr. Richard Muga, former director of Medical Services, that Oxford- and Cambridge-based scientists have used blood samples from the children to find an HIV vaccine, without the approval of the board. But no charges have been made against their care of the children, HIV-positive children who are staying alive. Children like Humphrey.)

We visited Humphrey a few times over the next few weeks, as Kevin would come down to Nairobi for brief periods on several occasions so as not to miss too much school at any one time. Kevin met Humphrey's nurse, the man who administered his medicines. He explained that the three different medicines

Humphrey took were all antiretroviral drugs, but all different classes of drugs, all fighting the virus. While this combination of drugs worked for Humphrey, what worked for him might not work for another child. He also talked about how some of the drugs needed refrigeration, which made it difficult for people in the rural areas both to have access to and store them. One of the medicines that he had was made by pharmaceutical giant Roche.

At the end, Humphrey and Kevin exchanged addresses, promising to write to each other. They clapped each other's hands with great gusto, and when we drove off, Kevin looked out the window much more pensively than usual.

Prior to our departure from Nyumbani, Father D'Agostino hadn't minced his words when it came to the pharmaceutical companies. He had called them "genocidal." We needed to talk to one of them: Roche.

CHAPTER TWENTY-SEVEN
WHO MAKES THE MEDICINES?

I would go to visit Christopher Murray and David Reddy of Roche at their headquarters in Basel, Switzerland. I had asked them Kevin's questions to begin with at the AIDS Conference, and they had appreciated looking at the AIDS epidemic through Kevin's eyes. So, when I asked if they would speak to me some more, even though they said they would normally have refused to be part of a film like ours, they agreed.

Veronica, my producer in Australia, had a sister living not far from Basel, in Zurich. There, her niece Julia, all of a gangly twelve, was doing a school project on AIDS orphans. Each child had to find some way they could be of help in the world. This was going to be Julia's way.

Julia learned about Kevin. She also learned about other children orphaned by the epidemic and wrote about them for her report. She was eager to meet Roche to see what they were doing about AIDS orphans, what they were doing about the AIDS epidemic, and how they were helping people like Kevin. We arranged to meet in Basel.

The absolute opposite of the disarray of Nairobi or Kisumu is Switzerland in general, and Basel specifically. It's an old city, with lovely stone buildings throughout the city center and the sturdy Rhine River running through the middle of the town, along which people promenade. I arrived on a Sunday in May.

Having worked with interfaith groups in Africa and elsewhere in the world, it was an interesting coincidence that I happened to wander past a church (in a city loaded with churches) on the one day of the year where there was an interfaith exhibit going on, teaching locals about the religions of the world such as Buddhism, Judaism, Hinduism, and Christianity.

Another coincidence was that Basel was also only a few kilometers from the Goetheanum, a building built according to the principles of Rudolf Steiner, whose Waldorf school I went to as a child and teenager in New York.

I had dinner with Christopher Murray of Roche that evening. The restaurant was in a leafy square, with older professional waiters in white suits—as far away from Kevin's chicken and French fries as one could get. (Chris did not pay for dinner. As we'd be filming him, that would obviously have been inappropriate, although spending Aussie dollars in Euros was expensive and I was heading toward broke again at the time.)

We talked about his wife and his now grown-up children. He had lived in Asia much of his life, and though he hailed from the United Kingdom, he'd been out of the country so long he wasn't sure he could ever live there again. He liked the peace and quiet of Basel, although he acknowledged it to be a bit dull compared to life in Asia. But being the director of Roche International—and thereby all the company's operations in the Middle East, Asia, and Africa—he still traveled a lot.

We talked about the AIDS epidemic. I got the sense he was genuinely concerned as a human being, and as a corporate citizen. Off the record, he was very outspoken against certain governments. On the record, he was still outspoken, blunt, to the point. He would like to see everybody who had AIDS treated. But, he admitted, he worked for a commercial organization. Commercial organizations had to make money.

I thought I had told him during the dinner that the next day he and David Reddy would be interviewed not by me, but by a twelve-year-old girl. I thought I had.

The next morning Julia and her mother drove in from Zurich. Julia was a reed-thin girl with almond-colored curls. She was at the age when she could not stand up straight but was always slouching this way or that, her hand in one pocket or the other, her yellow denim jacket draped over her.

She'd been doing a lot of thinking about AIDS, she said, and the plight of the orphans. As we drove toward the company headquarters, she told me that she used to play a fantasy of being an orphan. She would pretend to herself that her parents had died and that she had no one at all who cared for her. She could be very sad in this fantasy. The difference, she pointed out, was she could find her mother and father at the end of the fantasy and hug them or talk to them for real. Kevin couldn't do that. That struck her—the difference between fantasy and reality.

It reminded me of when I was her age. I had a similar fantasy of my parents dying. In mine, I think, they drove a car off a bridge into water. And my brother, sister, and I found ourselves all alone in the world. But . . . it turned out that my parents were actually very rich. They'd been pretending they were poor, keeping us in the small railroad flat above a carpet store on First Avenue, so we would understand. Understand what? The value of money.

Anyway, it was a fantasy.

We arrived at Roche and asked at the security desk for Christopher Murray and the woman from public relations whom we were supposed to meet.

The guard looked at us with the film equipment. That was not the problem. He pointed at Julia, and asked if we intended to take her upstairs with us.

Of course.

C'est impossible!

Chris and the woman from public relations came down. Chris seemed initially shocked to see Julia, so I mentioned that I thought we had discussed the previous night that the questions were all being asked by young people. He adjusted to the idea pretty quickly, however.

It was the security guard who had the problem.

Absolument. Non!

The insurance would not cover young people. We tried every one of the guard's supervisors in the book, but young people

135

could not go above the lobby. Something about secret labs. It was disappointing. Strange. Intriguing? Bizarre? But Julia was undaunted.

We could do the interview in the lobby?

No.

Finally Chris suggested the cafeteria, although it would be noisy. We didn't have a choice.

So we left the main building, Julia and Chris walking along the main road to the glass structure housing the cafeteria. Julia chatted to him animatedly about her concern for AIDS orphans, and he seemed genuinely taken with her. She seemed to kind of skip along, as they walked and talked.

At the cafeteria, amidst the various employees of this pharmaceutical company, Chris got a coffee and Julia an orange juice, then eventually they sat down and talked about orphans and AIDS. She asked what Roche were doing about orphans in particular. He replied that they were supporting an orphanage in Malawi.

Then she quite brightly asked him if he could make money with AIDS.

Chris told her that they could make money on AIDS drugs in the developed world, but in developing countries, no, they did not make money from AIDS. They gave the drugs away at cost. He said, "We are a commercial organization and all of the money that we invest into research and development comes from the profits that we make or the money that we make out of selling medication."

He said he thought the problem with AIDS was not just

keeping the drugs at a low or minimal cost (as activists and governments had been arguing) but also getting drugs and medical services to people, especially in rural areas. There simply weren't enough health-care workers. He also mentioned what Humphrey's nurses had told us, that some of the drugs needed refrigeration, again making it difficult to get them to the people in the countryside with no electricity.

Julia continued to question him, asking whether Roche couldn't do more. Toward the end, he said this to her, "The area I get very frustrated with is when people say that the pharmaceutical industry as a total isn't doing enough. You know, without the pharmaceutical industry all of the people who have AIDS today would have died."

We then went to meet David Reddy, HIV franchise leader, heading up the research into HIV drugs. Since we couldn't go into the headquarters to film him, either, we filmed Julia and him sitting on the floor in a wing of the art galleries sponsored by Roche. She explained to David how thinking about the AIDS orphans made her feel very sad.

He told her he felt sad, too. That this disease was unique, because of the fear it engendered in people. "I think with AIDS, with HIV, it's stronger than in any other disease that we've known, at least in our lifetime."

"How did it get this bad?" she asked.

"AIDS went unnoticed for decades in Africa, and by the time it was noticed, it took everybody too long to get working on it. And that's what's made the situation as bad as it is today."

Julia told him how she knew from watching the footage of

Kevin all about the stigma people had with HIV in Africa. David told her people still experienced stigmatization in the West as well. He told her a story about a friend of his, a woman with HIV/AIDS. Most people didn't want to drink from the same glass as her because of their fear of getting the virus. But his friend said she was scared of drinking from their glasses. They might have a common illness that her immune system, ravaged and under attack, wouldn't be able to take. Rather than we being afraid of her, she was afraid of us. David, even though he was a top researcher in his field, hadn't thought of it like that himself before.

He told Julia that, although there was no cure, at least the disease was treatable now in the West. He had friends who'd survived twenty years on drugs. He was proud of the fact that, of the four classes of ARVs, Roche had invented two. However, despite the medical advances, prevention was still the best option.

So twelve-year-old Julia and he agreed that condoms were a good idea.

At one point, Julia asked him to explain the virus. David described how it attacked a cell, and then that cell took over other cells, until we had no more defense systems left to fight it or any other disease.

Julia said it sounded like a video game of alien invaders.

Only the alien invaders were the virus.

CHAPTER TWENTY-EIGHT
WHAT JULIA DID AFTERWARD

We had lunch with David Reddy and then both he and Christopher Murray had long good-byes with Julia. She told them she was going to give a presentation to her class, to encourage them to help AIDS orphans, just as she was trying to help Kevin. They asked her if she would send them her presentation when she was finished.

They seemed touched by her.

It is my experience that no matter what our jobs, when it is a child talking to us about other children who are dying or who have no one to care for them, we get touched. We drop some of the concerns that we take for granted: how high our stocks must go, how we need low interest rates to keep our mortgages down, how we must toe the corporate line.

Julia sent what she thought the two men from Roche's answers were to her questions:

ROCHE INTERVIEW QUESTIONS AND ANSWERS

Q: What are you doing to stop AIDS?
A: We (ROCHE) develop drugs for AIDS.

Q: How did it get this bad?
A: They didn't know how quickly it was spreading.

Q: Why do you help people with AIDS?
A: Because we can.

Q: Can you make money from AIDS drugs?
A: Yes, but we don't make money in Africa.

Q: What do AIDS sufferers need to be treated with?
A: Drugs and respect.

Q: Why can't you look on the positive side and fix things now?
A: We try to so things don't get so bad.

Q: What are you doing to help AIDS orphans?
A: We are giving powdered medicines and supporting groups
   that can give them love.

Q: How can we (you) make a difference?
A: Raising awareness.

Q: How can I make a difference?
A: By talking to people and making them aware.

I was struck by one of Julia's questions when she'd been talking to David: "Why can't you look on the positive side?" She said she had read that by the year 2010 there would be twenty million orphans, so she'd asked David, "But we're not in the year 2010 now. So why can't we be positive?"

David hadn't understood; neither had I.

She went on as if it were obvious. It wasn't 2010 yet. It was 2005. So if we were positive and did something, there wouldn't have to be twenty million orphans.

Duh! as we used to say when I was a kid.

CHAPTER TWENTY-NINE

JUST HOW BAD IS THE AIDS EPIDEMIC?

In Nairobi, Kevin sat at Cathy's dining table, slouched in his red-and-black sweatshirt, which he kept on almost all the time. To him, Nairobi was cold. Compared to the baking heat of Kisumu, I suppose it was.

He watched Julia's interview and read the reports Julia had written on my computer. He was touched that someone far away in Europe wanted to ask these questions for him, for AIDS orphans. He harbored no animosity toward the pharmaceutical companies.

At this point, Kevin understood the AIDS epidemic as something that had hurt him and that was also impacting his community badly. But he didn't comprehend its global reach. His understanding was growing, however, as he'd started to digest the information from the AIDS Conference and now Julia's interviews with the same company that made the medicine Humphrey and his friends took.

But while they had improved, if people could get the medicine, did it always work?

Kevin and I had both seen individual people with full-blown HIV/AIDS. And in Malawi, I had gone to a hospital crowded with languid "TB" patients. The doctor there had said that, of course, all these TB patients would have HIV/AIDS, but that no one then was getting tested. "Then" was only two years earlier. I had also been to the Mombasa hospital where I'd met Jane Musyoka. But Kevin and I together had never seen a group of such patients and how they were cared for.

So, after many attempts, Cathy, Kevin, and I were given access to Mbagathi Hospital, in Nairobi, with the aid of the Ministry of Health. Still feeling a "chill," Kevin wore his red sweatshirt. The hospital was a group of single-story white buildings through which we were directed to the women's ward, a group of small rooms wedged in between two courtyards.

We met a nurse called Francis Otwane. Maybe in her mid-thirties, Francis was not a heavy woman but small and strong, her feet firmly planted on this earth. She had a set jaw, tired eyes, and a gentle but matter-of-fact demeanor. She offered to show us the patients in the clinic, and then Kevin could ask her his questions.

We followed her into the few rooms, barely able to look at the patients we passed.

"Hell on earth" is what newspapers always print in stories about war or earthquakes.

If those situations are hell, I don't know what to call what we saw.

One woman in a wheelchair was skin and bone.

Another woman had to wave away the flies from her face as they constantly attacked her diseased and almost shredded skin. She lay next to the window; one could only see her face; the rest of her was covered up in blankets.

Other women slept two to a bed, one person's feet at the other's head. Another woman was tied to her bed; one could only imagine why.

There were a few family members helping to spoon-feed some of the patients, who could not swallow the food as it dripped out of their mouths.

Kevin looked around, his face almost cut like stone. I wondered if this was too much for him. It felt like too much for Cathy and me, but I didn't allow myself to react yet. (That's the only thing one can do sometimes.)

We went out into the courtyard, and Kevin talked to Francis, away from the patients. She told him that, of the forty-five patients he had seen, forty of them were HIV positive. However, very few of them had been tested because they didn't want to know they had the disease. Because of the stigma. Still. And unless they volunteered to be tested, they could not be treated and would receive no medicines.

Kevin asked Francis if the antiretroviral drugs he'd heard about and seen Humphrey take always worked.

Francis replied, "They do. To some individuals. Some take those ARVs and within a lifespan of a few months, like three months, they improve. While others, once they take them, they develop complications. Their conditions worsen, and yet they die."

But, she repeated, if they would not take HIV tests voluntarily, there was little the hospital could do for them. Especially as it had such limited resources anyway.

Kevin asked her how it was being a nurse with AIDS patients.

Francis told him it was difficult. How it hurt to see these people suffer and die. She said, "Even if you are not infected yourself, we are affected so much. We feel moved."

Then Kevin's face melted. He spoke with a very big lump in his throat, and a face full of sorrow. "I also feel sad seeing them suffering. I feel very sorry for them. I wish to become a doctor also so that I can at least help."

She looked at him with her honest, forthright manner. She told him she hoped he would become a doctor.

CHAPTER THIRTY
HOW DID IT GET THIS BAD?

How did it get this bad? Julia had asked. Didn't anyone realize what was happening?

(And how would Kevin get to be a doctor?)

In search of answers to these questions, we went to speak to Professor A. B. C. Ocholla. (No, he was not named for Abstain, Be faithful, Condomize, but wouldn't say what the ABC stood for.) An anthropologist, he had been studying the epidemic since the '80s. His office was at the University of Nairobi.

To study at this university was Kevin's dream. It was the be-all and end-all from his perspective in Kisumu.

We walked through the entrance's stone arch onto campus. Kevin all of a sudden became very self-conscious, making sure none of the university students was looking at him as we filmed him. I asked him why he was suddenly nervous now, but he didn't reply and just walked on quickly. He had actually never been to a university campus before. Perhaps he didn't want to call attention to himself here, in case someone remembered years later!

We inquired as to where the anthropology department was, and Prof. Ocholla's office. And we finally found it, after getting lost in various different stairwells.

The professor was a distinguished-looking man in his sixties, with a gray beard, a friendly face, and a pronounced paunch in a light green shirt. His office was large, but overwhelmed by an anarchy of books and pamphlets, some in various positions and on shelves, and some creating a varied landscape on his desk.

He welcomed Kevin effusively, offering a seat to him. I told him how Kevin longed to go to the university, especially medical school. He asked Kevin about his grades, which Kevin admitted weren't as good as they had been before. They had a good talk, a fatherly, kind one, before getting to the central issue. Did anyone know the AIDS epidemic would get so bad?

Yes, the professor said. He did. He came around to Kevin, dragging a huge old dark green book. It was a book he had cowritten. In it were studies and maps of the different areas of Kenya he had done as far back as 1986. At that time, he emphasized, he had predicted to the Kenyan government just how bad the epidemic would get in Kenya.

(The professor was not alone in his predictions. Panos, a United Kingdom-based organization, also in 1986, had predicted how bad the epidemic would get in Africa, as did many other organizations. Unfortunately, as shocking as the predictions seemed then, the reality was invariably worse.)

Professor Ocholla said he and others had told the Kenyan government they had to take serious action. But because of the nature of the disease, because of the corrupt Moi dictatorship government, because of the priests who battled A. B. C. Ocholla on the condom issue, because, because, because . . . the disease ran rampant, especially where Kevin lived in Kisumu.

He gave one example of how around Kisumu the old practice of wife inheritance also contributed. If a man dies, his wife will marry his brother. The professor explained this was originally meant to ensure that the wife and her children would be taken care of within the family. But with husbands with HIV infecting their wives, then dying, and then the wives infecting their new husbands, the epidemic was compounded.

He had battled the previous Catholic archbishop, who had accused him of encouraging the youth to have sex by promoting condoms. Like Thailand's Senator Mechai, A. B. C. Ocholla had earned the nickname Mr. Condom.

Kevin, still worried about condoms after all this time, asked him about the new preventative methods of circumcision and microbicides. In the future, they seemed good to Ocholla. But only then—in the future.

Kevin just nodded. He promised to do better at his studies.

CHAPTER THIRTY-ONE

A NEW KIND OF "MISERY"

As we walked away from the professor's office and onto the university campus, I wanted to get a shot of Kevin gazing happily at his dream for the future. But Kevin was still so nervous of what these other people might think, even though he liked the idea of the shot, too, that he kept shuffling around, hemming and hawing. It reminded me of all the many times I had been too nervous to be "different" in front of other people, complete strangers. I said that to Kevin and then told him that I had finally realized that most likely I would never see any of these people again. And what was wrong with being different anyway?

Intellectually, he got it. Emotionally, he didn't. He looked miserable.

I asked him if he had imagined what it would feel like to attend this university. He smiled.

"It would be wonderful, of course."

I said, "But you look miserable, so maybe it would be miserable. Would it be miserable?"

He couldn't help smiling.

"Awful?" I asked.

"No. Miserable," he replied.

"Just absolutely miserable?"

"Yes, miserable," he said with a very wide grin. "Very miserable."

From then on, "miserable" took on a new meaning for us. There was miserable—and then there was miserable.

CHAPTER THIRTY-TWO
DR. RICHARD MUGA

Another miserable day was when we got to meet Dr. Richard Muga. Dr. Muga had formerly been the head of all medical services in Kenya but is now the chairman of the National Council for Population and Development. He is a big, strong man, distinguished but kind-looking. In his leather-paneled office, he showed Kevin literature about the epidemic in Kisumu and other regions of the country. He, too, was from western Kenya, about one hour's drive from where Kevin lived.

He asked Kevin about his life, nodding as Kevin told him about growing up as an orphan. Kevin glossed over how poor he'd been, but Dr. Muga picked up on it. "I, too, grew up poor," he said. "And yet, I became a doctor. I became head of all medical services in Kenya."

Kevin was impressed.

He told Kevin that he, too, had been directly affected. "Even me, as a doctor, I lost two brothers to the AIDS epidemic."

Kevin asked him about abstinence versus condoms.

Dr. Muga smiled. He said he had a son a few years older than Kevin. His son was now, like Kevin, a Catholic. He and his son discussed and debated condoms, and Dr. Muga said he wasn't there to push condoms. But, "for us, AIDS is real. AIDS is devastating. And if there is any clue, any way of protecting oneself, we must go for it. It doesn't mean we are forcing people to use condoms. But we give people a choice."

He was angry at the current U.S. administration for emphasizing abstinence before marriage and not promoting condom use for the youth. He felt the epidemic was above religious belief as far as public policy was concerned.

Dr. Muga talked about people he admired: Thoraya Obaid at the UNFPA; Mary Robinson; and Jeffrey Sachs, the economist who had an economic model of a village in Kenya in the hopes of practicing methods that would eradicate extreme poverty. That village, too, was about an hour and a half from where Kevin lived. (Kevin was quite at the epicenter of it all!)

He listened to Dr. Muga very attentively, charmed by him and his logic: he was not telling people to have sex, but if they were going to have sex, to use protection. I could see Kevin's face and brain grappling with the concept. Ever since he'd met Humphrey, his certainty regarding "abstinence only" had been shifting. It would continue to shift through meeting people like Dr. Muga.

But most teenagers in Kevin's community didn't get to speak to this many people about condoms or abstinence. They mainly got to speak to advisers like Albert.

Perhaps, then, this book is meant for everyone who can only talk to an Albert—as well-meaning as he is.

CHAPTER THIRTY-THREE

WHO'S IN CHARGE?

A few days later, after using various connections, pleading, and calling constantly, we finally got through; as we filmed in downtown Nairobi, Cathy's mobile rang. It was our contact, Anthony Lundi, who had just spoken to the Minister of Health, the Hon. Charity Ngilu. She was willing to meet Kevin Sumba, the orphan from Kisumu, if we went to her office immediately.

We went to her office immediately.

Kevin was very nervous the whole way. If he wanted to be a doctor, there was no one more important to meet. And that was true, too, if we wanted to understand how his government was now tackling the AIDS epidemic nationally.

I had heard a lot about the minister. She was an outspoken woman. During my previous visit to Nairobi, nurses had gone on strike. Charity Ngilu had subsequently threatened to fire the lot of them. There was footage on the news of her crying in the hospital as she watched sick people getting little help because of the strike. The nurses were arguing they could barely live on their wages. (This has become a huge problem: nurses are lured overseas to America and Australia, where there is better pay and a shortage of nurses. So, in Africa, where the AIDS epidemic is expanding, the medical staff is . . . contracting.) The minister claimed they didn't have enough money in the health department as it was, and so couldn't possibly meet the striking nurses' demands. In this case, I had taken the nurses' side.

The minister, however, was currently being lauded overseas. She was making a radical suggestion: that medical services be socialized. This would mean free or very cheap medical care, such as in some European countries, Canada, Australia, and Cuba. A daring idea indeed for a country that barely had antiretroviral drugs the first time I visited.

The Ministry of Health is a tall white building, set off on its own. We raced into the building (when I say raced, Kevin was walking slightly faster than normal—remember, polé polé, never too fast in Kenya). And of course we rushed in, only to be shown into the waiting room.

As we waited—and waited—I spoke to two interesting businessmen who were also there. One was friends with the minister, and had helped Lundi set up our interview. The other had a children's orphanage in a rural village. They, too, supported Ngilu's efforts in making medicine more affordable. Kevin, too shy and nervous to speak with them, instead picked up a copy of *Time* magazine. The cover featured a picture of the new Pope.

Finally, we entered the minister's office. Ms. Ngilu was busy on the phone, but after concluding her call came over immediately, sitting on the sofa and patting the space beside her for Kevin to sit. She smiled at him very warmly indeed. This was not the tough woman I'd seen on television. Businesslike, dressed in a knitted gray skirt and matching top, she was imposing but gently spoken, and she approached Kevin with an almost maternal touch.

She asked him about himself. He told her he was an orphan who had come to ask her questions about AIDS. That he was seventeen. And that he wanted to be a doctor. She listened respectfully, compassionately. She, too, seemed touched by him.

He asked her about medicines for people with HIV/AIDS. She told him she did not have the resources for all the people who needed the medicines. Those who really needed it at the moment, direly, numbered about 200,000, she said. By the year's end they were hoping—hoping—to be able to give about 30,000 of these people the medicines. About one-seventh of the desperate people.

Kevin asked her about children. "Do orphans have the right for free medication?"

"We are now giving free primary health care and that is in the rural areas and in the slums," she said. She told him they were trying to give free health care to all the children. But what was most important to her was telling the children and young people about HIV prevention. "We really target youth because youth are the ones who are most now affected and infected by HIV/AIDS. And especially, Kevin, somebody like you who is not having some parental guidance."

They talked some more. He told her what the archbishop had said. I told her what Albert had said to Kevin, which he confirmed. I also told her what the U.S. congressman had said to me about Africans. The more she listened, the more incensed she became.

She was especially angry with the people in power in America telling Africans to abstain. Who were not talking about condoms. Who were pushing health policies backed by religious ideology, in her country. Where these policies were killing her youth. It was the children in Kenya, in Africa, who were getting sick, who were not using condoms.

"I promote condoms, because I know the youth are getting infected every day. So if I can get the youth to use condoms and not get infected, it is cheaper to prevent than to treat. And it's cheaper to have people stay alive than for me to tell them 'abstain.' And nobody, nobody, should deny one their right to use condoms or not to use condoms."

Kevin listened to her, somberly, as if she were declaring war. A war that affected him.

CHAPTER THIRTY-FOUR
THE WAR

There was a war going on inside Kevin.

On the one hand, there were many religious leaders telling him, "No matter what, do not use condoms." They were fighting for his soul. They were not ill-meaning people. They helped people who were sick. But they were "adamant," to use their own word, against condom use. There was no sex until marriage. Period. And there were more people, religious leaders from the United States, coming to preach this message, which had also been advocated in schools in southern states in America.

I'd met one such leader at the new U.S. embassy on the outskirts of Nairobi, far from the destroyed one downtown. I was waiting to get more pages put into my passport, so I could continue traveling to ask more of Kevin's questions overseas. I had just mentioned to Cathy before she'd dropped me off that we should talk with an evangelical Christian missionary here. Lo and behold, one sat down right next to me at the embassy. A big man from Texas, with heavy jowls, dressed in a white shirt and vest and blue jeans, he asked me what I was doing here. I told him about Kevin and my questions about AIDS.

He told me he was here on a mission about AIDS, too. He was spreading the word of God and Jesus. He was teaching ministers how to spread the word. "If we can get these people to abstain, we can stop this epidemic." To date, his ministry had been funded by people's donations, but he was now applying for U.S. federal funding. He seemed to sincerely believe what he was saying. He was on his way to Tanzania to spread the word, then would come back to Kenya. He was a busy man, constantly traveling these parts himself, he said.

I wondered how many Alberts would be reached by his message across Africa.

On the other hand, people like Richard Muga, Charity Ngilu, or Father D'Agostino were telling youth, like Kevin, that condoms were all right, that they were necessary to stop the spread of AIDS. And if one was going to be realistic—if the enemy was the virus—then one had to do whatever was necessary to stop it.

Abstinence or condoms. Abstinence or condoms. I thought we should explore a country that had managed to move beyond this debate. A country affected by the AIDS epidemic that wasn't telling people to abstain, but which instead was specifically advocating condom use.

Over Thai chicken panang curry made by Jim, Cathy's husband, which was rather spicy but to Kevin's liking, I told him that while he went back to school, I would take his questions to Thailand, the country where I had first asked his questions at the International AIDS Conference. Senator Mechai had said he'd be happy to give us more time and answer more of Kevin's questions.

As he finished the panang, Kevin did drink a large glass of water. Quickly. As surprisingly open to trying new foods as he was, the sauce was a bit too hot for him.

CHAPTER THIRTY-FIVE

PONLAPAT TAKES ON KEVIN'S QUEST

I had first been to Thailand as a naïve young man a few years out of college (as opposed to the naïve somewhat older one that I am now). It had been my first time in Southeast Asia. I'd landed with a friend in Bangkok, the capital, a city then where the taxis didn't have meters and you had to bargain your fare, in that, at the time, wonderful mess of an airport. I'd fallen in love with the country instantly, with its three-wheeled *tuk-tuks* puttering around the streets, with its glittery temples, with the famous Thai smile, and with *sanuk*, that sense of enjoying life. And of course the marvelous street food, people cooking on small mobile stalls, fragrant smells greeting you everywhere you walk.

I remember sitting with my friend on the street, drinking a fresh juice and eating pad thai, that lovely classic noodle dish, while debating George H. W. Bush's invasion of Panama. Now all these years later, I was going back yet again to Bangkok, where George W. Bush's policies were in the news. In order for countries to receive funding to fight HIV/AIDS (countries selected by the U.S. administration), they could not distribute condoms to prostitutes for them to protect themselves, and ultimately others, from the epidemic. Instead, sex workers were supposed to be encouraged to choose a different profession. It was like encouraging abstinence, only in a different form.

It reminded me of the Indian sex worker I'd interviewed at the AIDS Conference who'd said, "ABC is absolutely wrong. It can never work. This will actually harm sex workers doubly. They will become more vulnerable to infection. And secondly they will become more destitute and poorer. Sex workers exist because men come to women to buy sex."

Men came to women to buy sex in Bangkok, famous for Patpong Street and its prostitutes and Nana Plaza—even attracting "sex tours" from Europe and America.

But there are many other aspects to the city.

Though it had changed drastically over the years, in terms of its sky train, modernization, and an ever-larger middle class, Bangkok still had a charm absolutely its own. I was fortunate in that, for the AIDS Conference, Pierre, my producer and friend, had found me a fantastic hotel, called Reflections, where each room was designed by a different artist, each more colorful and stranger than the last. It was where I had stayed during flight stopovers in the past year as well, so I had got to know the two lovely owners: one Thai—and, like me, a former resident of Amsterdam—and one Swiss.

I had also stayed in touch with Senator Mechai and Roger Short, who had gone to university with Mechai (there are no coincidences in this story!).

Mechai's mother was Scottish and his father Thai. He had told me how his mother had explained to him that he was rich not because he was particularly clever or hardworking, but by birth and luck. So he had a duty to help others. Thus, in the 1970s, Mechai had started the Population Development Authority (PDA), a family-planning agency meant to help drag the poorest Thai out of poverty. PDA's influence grew, and its policies were adopted by the government. PDA promoted condoms as a method of birth control, so when the AIDS epidemic hit Thailand in the 1980s, Mechai's organization was, of course, right in place to promote condoms, in all kinds of ways.

Now, on this trip, the second with Kevin's questions and now some of Kevin's experiences, I was going to work together with a Thai television crew from the state broadcaster, Channel 11. They were coproducing the program with us. In exchange they would get to air the finished film as well. I had come full circle from my first visit years ago: now I was actually working in Thailand, and specifically Bangkok.

The producer from Channel 11 was called Sumonpan, a very self-possessed woman in her forties, with a gentle but forthright personality. She had produced quite a lot of television, especially sports. With Mechai's help, Sumonpan discovered three young people, two girls and one boy, who had been found by PDA and were interested in promoting AIDS awareness. Sumonpan and the crew met the three young people on a Saturday at an AIDS workshop, as I was flying in that night, and was to meet the three and select one of them on the Sunday.

The two girls were lovely and sweet, but very shy. They were each around fourteen. The boy, like Kevin, was seventeen. Also like Kevin, he was somewhat lean and gawky yet charming. He had lost his father when he was very young, so he was partially orphaned and had been raised in difficult circumstances by his mother and grandmother. He had a certain simple presence. He was very interested in Kevin's questions. His name was Ponlapat.

Ponlapat, for the entire time we filmed, always wore clean white school shirts, dressing eerily like Kevin when we'd first met. Like Kevin, he desperately wanted to go to university, but Ponlapat's dream was to become a computer engineer. Unlike in Kenya, secondary school in Thailand did not require tuition fees, but there were book costs and other expenses, for which his mother had to work hard to pay.

We went to Ponlapat's house to meet his mother and grandmother. His mother was probably not much older than myself, with a rounded but sensitive face and very gentle eyes. The grandmother had a wizened face but a patient smile and kind eyes, especially when they looked on Ponlapat. Both women seemed very tired. Mornings and through lunchtime, they transformed the front of their small house into a noodle stall, selling a variety of fresh noodle and pork soups. His mother said she had to make the stock from scratch from a leg of pork, starting early every morning.

I received a Thai cooking lesson, when I asked if I could have chicken with my noodles instead of pork. She looked at Sumonpan, the producer, as if I were crazy. How could I have chicken with pork stock? If you have chicken, you have chicken stock. Pork, pork stock. And so on. I promised to remember this and had a bowl. It was delicious.

In the afternoons, when there was no more noodle soup business, the mother and grandmother packed salt. Both would sit on the ground. The mother would take one of the big sacks of salt, cut open the bottom, and pour the salt into a large bowl. Bare-handed, she would individually pack little plastic bags of salt, which Ponlapat would often later deliver to stores to sell. Ponlapat also sometimes helped to seal the salt bags with a small laminating machine. The grandmother tied them up into pretty-looking bundles with red string. They did this for hours, literally, until dinnertime.

I asked why the mother didn't use gloves. It slowed her down was her reply. I winced, thinking how much it would hurt if she had a cut.

They lived hard lives. The salt-packing business was something they'd done with Ponlapat's father. But he had died seventeen years ago, shortly after his boy was born. Since then, mother and grandmother had carried on. Business was getting worse, because now there were competitors in the neighborhood. They had been forced to sell the house to make ends meet, now renting the home they had once owned. Their hope was that Ponlapat would do well.

His mother said she sometimes felt too cut off from Ponlapat. That she knew he was a teenager and educated now, and she a simple salt merchant. She looked as if she were about to cry.

At dinner, the three sat at a small table on the linoleum floor, sharing a small fish, rice, and some vegetables. As they ate, they watched the news on an old TV without speaking to each other.

After dinner, his mother went up to her room to pray at the family shrine. After Ponlapat cleared the food and table, his grandmother sat with him downstairs. She told him, "We haven't got much energy left. Don't get involved with drugs. Pay close attention to your studies. And don't go and get AIDS. Once you are afflicted, no one will take care of you. Isn't that right? Do you understand?"

Ponlapat went to see his mother. He prayed with her. Then she sat opposite him. She wanted to talk to him about how she felt. Perhaps this was only for our benefit, but she did cry. Tears came from her eyes and Ponlapat's as he listened to her. I looked from them to the picture of the young man that had been Ponlapat's father—not much older than Ponlapat was now when he died. His ghost seemed to haunt them all.

Ponlapat's mother said, "I have been taking care of you since you were three months, since your foot was as small as a clamshell. Don't forget that I am proud of you but you have to keep on. And come and consult me every now and then. Don't just go and do things as you like. Every day I work very tiredly, even when my hands are in pain from the salt. I am tired when I pack the salt, but I bear it. You have to try and make life better so when you grow up I can depend on you. We are in a difficult position, understand?"

We talked to Ponlapat in his room, adorned with posters of various Thai singers who were unfamiliar to me. Ponlapat told me about how he had been selected to do AIDS-awareness training due to his leadership in an antinarcotics training program and his coaching of junior students. He was very proud of being picked. I showed him footage of Kevin, including Kevin's conversations with Albert and the archbishop. Ponlapat was also religious, albeit Buddhist.

When I asked him for his impressions, he said, "Kevin is a person who is sad because he doesn't have both his parents. It's like me who has no father: I still have my mother. But Kevin is worse than me; he doesn't have both parents. It would be more difficult for him. But he is fortunate with respect to the fact he has some educational scholarship.

"I miss my dad, but if I were to have my dad at the moment my mum would not be in such a difficult position, because he would be making my family even more complete. I have only seen his pictures. I have never seen him in reality."

As far as his own AIDS-awareness training went, Ponlapat had been taught that condoms worked to prevent getting the virus. This is now what he was telling others in school. When he heard what Kevin had been told, he said, "If we don't use the condom and have sex with a person who has AIDS, then we would contract AIDS. Because sexual intercourse is the starting point of AIDS. I believe the archbishop has misunderstood something."

Over the course of our stay, we were going to see what other work Mechai's organization did, besides speaking at schools.

We were going to go with them to hand out free condoms at night to the prostitutes near the notorious Nana gallery. But Ponlapat wanted to bring some of his friends along. I wondered about the appropriateness of this, but Sumonpan said it was the way things were done. Thai youth did not go anywhere alone but always did things together. And so Ponlapat and his friends piled into the van with Sumonpan, the crew, and myself to drive into town.

We met up with the woman who was the AIDS training officer at PDA's headquarters, and then went to the Nana district, which was only a few blocks away. In an office there, Ponlapat's friends literally dressed up—a Mechai antic—as large colorful condoms, one green, one purple, another red. Then, as the endless variations of pumping music throbbed, and predominantly Western men checked out all the young Thai women, the officer and Ponlapat walked around, passing neon sign after neon sign: Pretty Lady, Red Lips, Cathouse, Pharaoh's.

From a small bucket, with his friends dressed as giant condoms behind him and the training officer, Ponlapat handed out condoms to the scantily dressed young women, who smiled or giggled as they took them from him. Familiar with the woman from PDA, they talked easily to Ponlapat, though he was nervous, having never been to a place like this before. Some of the girls were dressed only in bikinis; some in g-strings, and some were dressed as schoolgirls. The customers looked at Ponlapat oddly, and the Thai bouncers kept their stern faces on, making it clear that we should all move on rather quickly.

MILES ROSTON

Afterward, on the street outside, where the night stalls sold juices, fried fish cakes and basil, and pad thai, we could see the young women from a distance in the bars, chatting with their potential customers. But Ponlapat said, "I feel excited. This is a good campaign to stop AIDS from spreading. And these women who sell services—streetwalkers—this is the first time I've seen them. It's part of a campaign in which I can help. I treat it as offering help to the people. I'm not worried, as long as they know how to protect themselves."

Then he said something that touched me. "My feeling toward the women who offer services here is surprise. Because they are more or less the same age as I am. And also some of them would still be at school."

(A young Australian named Alex working at PDA later told me that U.S. officials who had long worked with the organization were no longer attending their meetings, because PDA was promoting condoms to these young women.)

On another evening, after school, Ponlapat and his friends, together with the headmaster, went to meet Senator Mechai himself. We went to his restaurant, Cabbages and Condoms. The garden was full of tables and lit by fairy lights. This was where Polnapat's friends waited. The place was rather famous in Bangkok, not necessarily for its food—which is good—but for its mission and the decor: the interior was decorated with condoms from every country in the world. A sign as we entered read: "Sorry, we have no mints. Please take a condom instead." Below that were two separate boxes: "Democrat size" and "Republican size." (Not surprisingly, it was Mechai who had

168

organized a "Cops and Rubbers" exhibit at the AIDS Conference the previous year!)

Ponlapat was understandably nervous about meeting the famous Senator Mechai and bowed to him very politely. (In Thai, the traditional bow with both hands clasped together is called a wai; it is a greeting to the Buddha nature in the other person.) Mechai bowed back, taking time out of his busy schedule of courting donors, endless meetings, policy decisions, and, now, being a grandfather, to talk to the young man.

Ponlapat said, "I would like to ask you, Khun Mechai, your opinion on the AIDS problem." (Khun is a respectful form of address.)

"Are you talking about Thailand or the world?"

"Of Thailand."

Mechai said, "It's better than before. New cases of people infected with AIDS have decreased by 90 percent. But AIDS is a universal problem. It happens in every country. And it is not only the problem of the Department of Public Health. It's everyone's problem. If everybody pays attention to it, then we'll understand how to prevent it. 700,000 Thai people have died of AIDS so far. There are another 700,000 who are surviving."

He said Thailand had been promoting condoms and safe-sex practices among the adults, and it had worked in decreasing the epidemic, which earlier on many had thought would spiral out of control.

But Mechai had a new fear, in line with what was happening worldwide. "The new cases consist mainly of teenagers. Because our government has been too quiet in distributing knowledge in schools. If schools don't spread the information, then students won't know much about AIDS. AIDS among youngsters is increasing each day. They must have factual knowledge or the problem will deteriorate."

"What solutions have you got for the problem?" Ponlapat asked.

"Most of the teenage cases are due to sexual intercourse. We must give them information about safe sex and how AIDS is spread. How to prevent it. We can't tell whether a person has AIDS or not by looking at them. So you must use a condom. Or, if you don't want the risk, don't have intercourse! But if you have sex, you should use condoms."

"Khun Mechai, what opinion do you have of the fact that Kevin's archbishop in Kenya advised Kevin and other teenagers not to use the condom in sex?"

Mechai took a minute before answering. "It is a pity that Kevin has been told not to use the condom. For teenagers who lose their life because of AIDS, will this archbishop be willing to take responsibility? All I can say is if we have more preachers of this type, then the world will be a worse-off place. In the next life, if you need to meet this preacher again, you can go and see him in hell. You won't find him in heaven."

Mechai's tone was, to quote the archbishop, adamant.

Senator Mechai did, however, see religion having a strong role to play in caring for people and making sure their rights were upheld, whether they were patients or children orphaned by the epidemic. "One more thing that we must do for people who have contracted AIDS, we need to take care of them. Don't let them be despised by society. And in Thailand the government has medication for everyone. With medication, you can prolong life ten or twenty years. Thai society should acknowledge that HIV-positive people should not be despised. We cohabitate with them."

After talking together, Mechai showed Ponlapat around the restaurant, pointing out the condoms on the wall and the painting of the Mona Lisa holding a lemon—a tribute to his friend Roger Short's project of lemon juice as a microbicide.

Then all the boys (and the crew) had dinner outside in the garden.

Just as the Catholic Church had its Nyumbani orphanage among other institutions to care for people, so Buddhists had set up care for people affected by AIDS. One of these institutions was Wat Prabat Nampu, a hospice for people in the last stages of the disease and also an orphanage, set up by the Buddhist monk Dr. Arthorn Prachanat. We decided to see for ourselves how the patients and children were being cared for, though both were hours away.

Of course, Ponlapat insisted on bringing at least one of his friends. What he didn't tell us was that his friend hadn't asked permission from his father. We were already a hundred or so kilometers into our trip when the friend's father called Sumonpan, furious that we had "absconded" with his son. He was yelling down the line.

Sumonpan listened patiently—patience is very much her virtue—before explaining that there was no turning back.

We passed the ancient city of Ayutthaya, with its dramatic

decaying stone ruins, and monkeys playing in its mist, then eventually reached the rural areas, with the almost neon green of rice paddies and beautiful old dark brown Thai teak houses.

At the entrance to the hospice, Ponlapat bowed to the Buddha atop the hill then entered the compound. We found the head nurse, a very kindly man, who offered to take us around. Inside, just like the hospital in Kenya, were many people basically on what might eventually be their deathbeds. But it was a much larger and cleaner hospital than what we'd seen in Kenya, with individual beds for patients, and even a bit of space around them. The nurse explained that, despite appearances, some of these men and women did get better on the antiretroviral drugs, and surprised even themselves by recovering.

One woman sat and watched us, emaciated and thin, but proud, very proud. She reminded me of Jane, who had looked at Kevin with very much the same eyes.

Unlike Kevin, Ponlapat was able to muster the strength to speak to the patients. But then he had not been impacted by AIDS in the same way Kevin had; he hadn't seen it up close before or been so personally affected by it.

Ponlapat talked to a gaunt gentle-looking man, maybe in his thirties, who told Ponlapat he was homosexual. He wasn't that sick now—he had responded well to the medicines—but he was here because he didn't want to be a burden to his family. He felt discriminated against back home. Not because of his sexual orientation, but because of AIDS. People were scared of him and didn't want to care for him. He said it was much better to be in this hospice provided by the monks. It was evident that Mechai was right: there was still a lot of stigmatization in Thailand, too.

Ponlapat listened attentively, giving a willing ear to this man. I liked Ponlapat more and more; he seemed truly a young man who was interested in other people, open and nonjudgmental.

Also in the hospice was a young woman, very far gone into the disease. A thin white man in his late fifties with black plastic glasses was leaning over and talking to her. We came over to see her. She had lost so much weight her breasts had wasted away to nothing, and she no longer had the strength to sit up. The older man held her hand encouragingly. She said she still liked to sing. The man told us, in an American accent that I felt I recognized, that she was a beautiful singer. Did we want to hear?

She began to sing to us. Lying on her back, she sang a very beautiful Chinese traditional song, but she sang it in Thai. Ponlapat listened, nodding his head to the beat. Tears welled up in my eyes. She looked from him to me, and back again. She was indeed a beautiful singer.

As Ponlapat talked with her, I spoke with the man caring for her. He told me he understood she had been a cabaret singer in Bangkok before she had become ill. He was impressed by her remarkable courage in the face of the disease, especially as she had not responded to the medication.

I asked him where he was from, saying his accent sounded very familiar. His name was Michael, Father Michael, a Catholic originally from the Bronx, where my father, also named Michael, grew up. This Father Michael was now living here to exchange understanding with the Buddhists, to help and care in whatever way he could. He said he got far more from the patients than they got from him in terms of learning understanding and patience.

When we took our leave of the young woman, she held our hands softly, but still with a little bit of grip, a grip holding onto life. She and Father Michael looked at each other with what looked to me to be real companionable love and compassion—both of them.

Afterward, we got into the van to drive to the orphanage, I saw Father Michael ride away on a rickety old black bicycle. He waved, as he rode into a rice field, a thin figure a long way from the Bronx but, I thought, very close to home.

CHAPTER THIRTY-SIX

THE SOUND OF ONE HEART BREAKING

We arrived at the orphanage of Wat Prabat Nampu, the facility founded by Dr. Prachanat. There were large institutional buildings on one side (which turned out to be schools and the hospital). On the other side were smaller cottage-type buildings, with green roofs and white walls; while in the center were free spaces, grass with open pagodas to sit in. There was also a lovely store in the middle where all the kids would shop for candy, sodas, crushed-ice drinks, little toys, and odds and ends.

Although not all of the children there were HIV positive, many were. Some were also orphaned.

We walked and talked with a few of these children, guided by the trainees, men and women in their early twenties, who were taking care of them. We went into the hospital, where we saw a tiny child who was incredibly weak, emaciated, barely able to sit up. Ponlapat talked with him and told him it would get better. The boy must have been all of five or six.

On the porch we found some healthier children. They laughed and danced; they pulled funny faces at the camera, some with huge marks on their skin. Many of them had been at the orphanage a while, but none of them had reached adolescence like Humphrey. At least now their medications seemed to be working, we were told. This facility was new, and had only taken the young children for the time being.

A young boy with boils all over his small body was sitting all alone on the grass. Ponlapat went to talk to him. He had been brought to the orphanage that day. The little boy could barely reply "yes" or "no" when Ponlapat spoke to him, then just held his hand. We bought him a candy bar, which Ponlapat gave to him. Though that didn't necessarily cheer him up, he did eat it.

The girl who really broke our hearts was Pin. Pin was maybe ten years old. She was an orphan from the north we were told, and when she began to get sick, her aunt could no longer care for her. She had a shoulder-length black bob of hair, and a downcast but very pretty face with beautiful light almond-brown skin. We bought her a crushed-ice drink with sweet lemon syrup. She sipped on it as she and Ponlapat sat in one of the pagodas and talked. For the most part, it was Ponlapat doing the talking.

He asked, "Where are your parents?"

"They all passed away."

"Do you miss them?"

"I miss them."

"If you had your parents with you, wouldn't it be better?"

"Yes."

"It's like me," Ponlapat said. "I haven't got my father as well. When did your parents pass away?"

And this is what she said: "On Wednesday."

"Can you remember which year?"

She couldn't.

"Since your parents passed away, who did you go and live with?"

"I lived with my auntie."

Her auntie delivered her here. Because she needed medication. She needed medical care.

"Do you miss your parents?"

"Yes," she said emphatically.

"What do you do when you miss them?"

She took a moment. "I cry."

She told him she was very lonely.

Lonely. Kevin was lonely.

"What dreams do you have for the future?"

"I want to become a nurse."

"What do you think about being a nurse? Is it good?"

She nodded. "When I was sick with dengue fever, I was helped by a nurse."

She was still very sad, and Ponlapat wanted to cheer her up. So he asked if she had a favorite song. She did.

"My favorite song is the 'Carrot Song.'"

Ponlapat asked if she would sing it for him.

She smiled, a gasp of a smile, for the first time. She stood up and began to sing.

They are the carrot farmers
I come to school early in the morning
and the carrot farmers kindly bring along those carrots
eating carrots makes you look good.

Then Pin began to dance.

And it has vitamins
Your cheeks will be red
Because you eat carrots
You are a young student with a small body
You use the fan and you also have wind blowing against
you
And there is a cool breeze blowing.

Then she stopped, after doing a little jig of a dance. "That's all I can remember." She sat down, pleased with herself.

We went to the little store and bought a lot of little toys and candies for her. She deserves so many little toys and candies and big toys and candies. All the children there do. And as many crushed-ice drinks with sweet lemon syrups as their hearts desire.

CHAPTER THIRTY-SEVEN
LORD BUDDHA AND CONDOMS

It was dark, dinnertime, so Pin went off to eat. Ponlapat had one more thing to do here. He was going to talk to the man responsible for building this orphanage, the Buddhist monk Dr. Arthorn Prachanat. Ponlapat, a Buddhist like most Thais, wanted to know firsthand what his religion said about condoms.

Dr. Prachanat, a smiling man of indeterminate age—perhaps in his midfifties—arrived in a white van, wearing his orange robes. He and Ponlapat sat on the steps overlooking the whole facility in the dark. Ponlapat bowed to him, and they began to talk.

Ponlapat began by saying, "I would like to know why would a monk want to come and help in the problem of AIDS."

"Well, when the AIDS epidemic started in Thailand about twenty years ago, because of a lack of knowledge, the Thai people were afraid of it and despised those who had it. A person afflicted with AIDS would be deserted by the family as well as by the society. This included the care of patients in the first era [the early days of the epidemic]. Even the doctors and nurses were afraid of them. The patients were ostracized and chased away from their own homes fifteen years ago. Then the Thai temples got more information about AIDS, and people afflicted started to seek refuge in the temples."

He said that at first the monks hadn't even known what the people were sick with, but they knew the patients had the right to be treated with dignity, had the right to medicine.

Ponlapat asked, very earnestly, if there was any clear indication in Buddhism about how to take care of AIDS patients.

Dr. Prachanat answered, "When we talk about the AIDS epidemic, this is something new. Even for Buddhist teachings, the epidemic is a new thing. But when we are talking about Buddhism, whatever type of sickness, the Lord Buddha himself taught that, if we take care of sick people, it is like taking care of the body of the Buddha himself. Therefore Thai people like to give alms to the sick people or those approaching death. We like to give alms at the hospital, at the elderly residences. Take, for example, at Wat Prabat Nampu [which Ponlapat had just visited] where there are a lot of AIDS patients living, there are a lot of people who come to make merit, to give alms there to the patients so that they can have medication, food, clothing, and other necessities. If we refer to the principles of our religion, this is an important thing, because coexistence relies on the greatest dharma principle [the principles of Buddha's teaching], and that is to have compassion."

Finally, Ponlapat brought up Kevin. He said Kevin had been receiving lessons from his preacher that he must not use a condom if having sexual intercourse. What was the Buddhist teaching about this?

And Ponlapat's monk said, "You must understand that the use of condoms prevents conception. Originally, there wasn't such a thing called contraception. During the era of the Lord Buddha, there weren't any condoms at all. It would have been less than one hundred years ago that people started making it possible for people to have sexual intercourse without conception."

Ponlapat asked, "You mean not having children?"

"Yes, not having children. If you ask me what does Buddhism say about this matter, well, I can tell you Buddhism emphasizes the way of nature. Which means that when a woman is ready to conceive and then has sexual intercourse, it then becomes a part of nature for her to bear any number of children. All that is required is that the person is ready and prepared to take care of the new life that came into being. That's a good thing.

"But when the population of the world increased to an extent, people started to find ways to slow down the growth. So they are increasing ways of preventing conception, making each family to have perhaps only two or three children. Our grandparents used to have more than ten children. Because we did not have any prevention of conception.

"But if you ask me whether the use of a condom is wrong, well, considering the population and public health, it is not wrong. In Buddhism we do not forbid people from using it.

Neither do we promote its use. Because we haven't been stating this anywhere from the beginning."

The drive home that night was long. Ponlapat's friend was worried about what his father would do when he got home.

So was Sumonpan.

We stopped for dinner at the Thai equivalent of a truck stop, only we got to enjoy fresh beef with chilies, lovely pork noodle soups (which the crew had—not Ponlapat who could have that at home), and Sumonpan and I shared a large Singha beer. We both needed it.

When we stopped for gas, I asked Ponlapat how he had found his visit to the hospice and orphanage. Ponlapat said he had been moved, as this was the first time he had got to meet people with HIV/AIDS. "I have sympathy for them, and yet am also excited because this is the first time I am able to meet them. And I was able to meet orphans who had contracted AIDS. And these youngsters, some of them are still strong physically. But some of them have scars all over their body. I pity them. I want to tell junior students in my school to be aware about AIDS. When you are young, to learn the importance of the various protective methods. So that when you grow up, you can use them."

We were all quiet for the rest of the drive home. I kept thinking about the Buddhist monk's words about condoms "considering the public health."

I also kept thinking about little Pin. I noticed that Ponlapat had a tear in his eye at one point. His friend and his friend's father would be all right. It was the children without fathers— and mothers—we needed to worry about.

When he arrived home, as was customary, Ponlapat prayed to the shrine.

In my hotel room at Reflections, I prayed, too. I just didn't know to whom.

CHAPTER THIRTY-EIGHT
KEVIN AND HIS RIGHTS

The stories from Thailand, of patients being discriminated against, of people having to take refuge because of having HIV/AIDS, of young people suffering because they had the disease or their parents had it, were not really new to Kevin. What was new to him was that they were happening, had happened, in another place halfway around the world, where they liked their food spicy, and only ate chicken and French fries on the odd occasion when they might go to KFC.

What Kevin didn't have that even Pin, the poor little girl in the Buddhist orphanage had, was anyone to care for him. Ann and Evelyn had Lucy Yinda. Humphrey had Father D'Agostino.

The more time I spent with Kevin, the more I realized how much of an issue this was. I had been told that keeping him in his community was the best thing for him, but what community?

To me, a non-African from thousands of miles away, it was just starting to seem cruel that he had to live alone. And I felt responsible for his plight, too. I thought back to his original questions. These were a few of the things he had written: "How and what responsibilities will they take to ensure those affected live longer and lead a normal life full of happiness and not sorrow and suffering? What responsibility will they take to ensure that those left do not suffer much, especially orphans?"

What he was talking about were his rights. Did he have any? What were they?

The first time we'd explored this concept together was in Kisumu on my first trip back in November 2004. We'd met with a woman named Frida, who was the local child rights counselor. She had an office at another Catholic Centre. She was a very sweet and, for a rights advocate, a very soft-spoken woman. She and Kevin had sat down and talked, and I am not sure exactly what happened but it literally became a comedy of errors—if the word "comedy" can be used in such a case.

She told him that her organization often advocated for children whose property had been stolen. He listened intently. She told him that children's relatives often stole their inheritance— their land, their valuables—when the parents died.

Kevin then said he had had his property, his land stolen.

I was shocked. I'd always understood that his mother had lived in the same shack he lived in now, and that there was no rural home or property left. (Many Kenyans may live in abject poverty in the cities, but do have a small family property in the rural areas. But all Kevin's uncles, aunts, and grandparents had passed away, with the exception of that one poor uncle up north in Eldoret.)

Frida proceeded to explain to Kevin how they could go to court and sue his relative to get the property back. She started asking questions about his property. I tried to interrupt as he began to tell her about someone who had stolen his land. Frida just shushed me.

Later, I asked Kevin if what he'd said was true. He said no. I asked him why he'd made up all those things about his property, then. He shrugged; he'd thought it would make the conversation more interesting. He was acting—for her, for us, for the camera. (Remember, this was before he'd seen *Star Wars!*)

Many months later, Kevin took a few days off school again, and this time flew down to Nairobi, emerging from the small domestic airport terminal looking very ill, accompanied by Frederik, who had meetings in the capital and had kindly offered to fly down with the boy. Later, when Kevin had recovered from his airsickness, and had had some tea and toast, we drove to the offices of The Cradle.

Here we met with Millie Odhiambo. Millie is the founder of this organization in Kenya, which works to uphold children's rights. They operate in Kenya and also work with other organizations around the continent. She is a striking woman, with a very high forehead and high head of hair, and a strong presence. We met her at her offices, which were simple and unadorned.

Kevin asked her how he could protect his rights.

"First," she said, "you have to know what your rights are." She explained to him that the Kenyan government had actually guaranteed many things in a Child Rights Act. That Kevin had a right to medicine. He had a right to food.

He also had a right to go to school. Parents had to guarantee their children an education. "One of the things that the law provides very specifically is that children have a right to education, and that duty falls on the parents and the government. So in a situation where the parent is not there, then the government must come in and take control."

Kevin was confused. How come he needed a charity to pay his secondary school fees if he had the right? How come he hadn't known about any of this?

Millie explained that just because there was a Child Rights Act, it didn't mean that any of its provisions were enforced. Children were not supposed to be locked up without due process, yet in practice they were constantly. And one of the roles of Millie's organization was to defend them.

She told him about one new right and what was happening with that. It was called a bursary fund. The bursary fund was supposed to help poor children, particularly orphans of AIDS, with their school fees. Kevin grew excited. But Millie said the amount would be only about 10 percent of the fees. Still, it was something, a start. But then came the zinger. "What happens instead is some members of parliament actually use that fund to give to maybe their friends or their relatives."

In Millie's mind, the problem in Kenya was not just lack of money, because there were quite a few people making lots of money. The problem was what people did with that money. Corruption was rife, and this was one incredibly blatant example of that. (All one had to do was read the various local newspapers to get a sense of just how much corruption there was. It was a daily item, just like the promotions to glory in the obituaries.)

Millie explained that some members of parliament would just put forward their own names, their friends' children's names, perhaps the names of the people who voted for them. Et voilà, disappearing bursary funds.

Disappointed, Kevin asked her if the AIDS epidemic made the plight of orphans worse.

Of course, she said. Because of the AIDS epidemic there were now so many more orphans. And so many of them wound up on the street. "It is not just about you, Kevin. There are so many orphans. There are so so many orphans and not just in Kisumu, but if you walk even in the streets of Nairobi, you'll see so many children that have come to the streets because of the problems that they are facing."

Through the good graces of Anthony Lundi (who knew Millie, and who had hooked us up with Health Minister Charity Ngilu), we did get to meet some of these street children in Nairobi.

I have had many sleepless nights since then.

Anthony Lundi used to work in the government. Now he was running a program, overseen by the vice president of Kenya, Dr. Moody Awori, attempting to build schools for street children and get them off the streets. The program had come under intense pressure. Members of parliament wanted to know why money was being spent on building schools for these chil-

dren when there were so many other schools to be built for just
the primary schoolchildren who had families. Remember, under
the new government, primary school education was now free,
but that meant they actually had to have schools to send the
children to. And teachers and . . .

We knew that to meet any of these street children, we had to
go with someone they knew and trusted. Nairobi was full of stories of drugged-out street children throwing battery acid
through car windows at drivers, and other such dangers. The
children were supposed to be high on glue and have no regard
for human life.

So Anthony and his team led Kevin, Cathy, and me to the
river. I had not even known there was a river running through
the city. But there was, perhaps a fifteen-minute walk from
downtown Nairobi.

Near the banks of the river, as the area grew ever more
squalid, and garbage-strewn, we met with one of the leaders of
the children, a guy perhaps in his early twenties, haggard,
tough, scraggy. He gave his word to Lundi that we'd be fine.
And as Lundi was trying to help the kids, the man seemed to
trust him. We followed him, and were immediately surrounded
by these "children."

I use quotation marks because at first I could not see them
as children. They appeared to me like creatures. Not children.
Some of them wore plastic bags; some wore newspapers as
clothing. A few wore torn pieces of woven cloth that may
have once been sweaters. Their skin was blotchy, dirty; mucus
ran from their noses. They were high, rambling, too excitable,

violent, and unpredictable, as they sniffed glue from under their sleeves, sniffed glue from plastic bottles.

We followed them to where they lived, by this "river." This was not the Hudson. This was not the Seine, the Thames, or the Rhine in Basel where Roche was. It was not the pretty Yarra running through Melbourne. The river had literally become a garbage dump. And right beside it, on the mounds of refuse, is where these "creatures," coated with dirt, dressed in rags or old newspapers, lived.

The air that day, I remember, was gray, thick with smog. Kevin stood, not terrified, but stunned. Finally, a few of the children talked to me. I remember one in particular, who became ever more human in my eyes as he came up to me and spoke, and that realization almost hurt too much. He kept motioning as if he were writing with one of his hands on his other hand, and talking, almost sobbing. When I asked Lundi what he was saying, he told me the boy was saying he wanted to go to school.

This world was like the night of the living dead. Only it was daytime. And real.

Most of these children—for they were not creatures, after all—were between eight and, say, fourteen. An older boy came by all of a sudden with a box. And in the box was a small boy. The older teen, maybe Kevin's age, put the box down, and the little boy came toward us, his arms outstretched. If that boy was older than three, I'd be shocked. He, too, was living on this garbage dump.

Kevin talked to some of the children. More and more circled

around us. Just the sight of the camera made them more excitable. They were absolutely high as kites, crowding in on us. Lundi said we should leave, as they would soon go out of control. Understandably. But one could feel their hunger, their glue-fed craziness rising.

We left, giving the leader some money for them as we walked away.

If *I* had to live on the street like these children, I would be sniffing glue morning to night.

Kevin said to me later, "They sniff glue because they don't want to feel anything. The street children don't have school. They want to go. They are children. They don't have food. The place they live is terrible. If I didn't have the support of my neighbors, who knows if I would have been on the street?"

I look at my photos of these children to remind myself sometimes. To remind myself of what? In the photos, there's the back of Kevin's head, and two boys probably about fourteen sniffing glue and acting proud, standing on a heap of garbage. In another one, there's a boy with a glue bottle literally up his nose, in an old overcoat. His eyes look dead.

I look at these images to remind myself that no one, on this planet or any other, should have to live the way these children do.

Millie had said they had rights. What rights? What rights did Kevin have?

CHAPTER THIRTY-NINE
HUMAN RIGHTS

If Kenya, and other local countries, were not guaranteeing Kevin's and these street children's rights, who was? What would the international organizations and their leaders pledged to protect these children say?

I went back to New York, my birthplace and of course the headquarters of the United Nations. I went to meet up with Carolina, whom I'd first met and asked Kevin's questions of at the AIDS Conference. I had taped Kevin's new specific questions for her and the leaders she would meet, leaders whom Pierre, my producer in the United States, had set up for us to interview. Carolina would meet Mary Robinson, from the AIDS Conference, perhaps the foremost authority on human rights as the former UN Commissioner of Human Rights; as well as two other leaders in the worldwide fight against HIV/AIDS whom Dr. Richard Muga had told Kevin about: Jeffrey Sachs and Thoraya Obaid.

It turned out that this was also the same week as Carolina's high school prom—an event a world removed from that of the street children.

Carolina's father was Mexican, her mother Nicaraguan. And she had grown up in Nicaragua and then Peru. Both her parents were journalists, very much leaning to the left. In Peru, her father had been the first to make contact with the guerrillas who had hijacked the Japanese embassy and everyone in it in Lima for months during 1996–97—a huge story at the time. Though it should have done wonders for his career, it made him a target for the government, as they claimed he was enabling the hijackers. He sent his family to the United States, where his wife was now working for CBS, and then escaped himself. Now, he was freelancing as a cameraman.

The family lived in a nice suburb in New Jersey, with Carolina attending what was supposed to be one of the top ten schools in America. And Carolina had become . . . a football cheerleader. Yes, with pom-poms and the short-skirt outfits. She was so dedicated to it that she even went to football cheerleading camp in the summer. She was becoming more all-American than an all-American could be.

Which is probably why her mother and father had taken her and her brother along to the AIDS Conference in Bangkok—for a dose of international reality. Carolina had been moved, almost shocked, by what she had seen there. As she said, she'd had no idea AIDS "was a big deal."

Pierre and I met her again in New York. We had lunch with her and her mother at a restaurant on Sixth Avenue. The memory of the AIDS epidemic had faded a bit for her, until I played her the video of Kevin now on my computer. She watched, rapt, the video playing back reflected in her eyes. When she finished, she told us about her return from the AIDS Conference. Her friends had asked her if she hadn't been scared to meet someone with AIDS there. Wasn't she frightened that she could have caught the disease—just by meeting them? And at a meeting of cheerleaders' parents, her mother was told they were shocked that she would let Carolina go to something like that. These were parents and students from a top-ten public school in the United States of America.

Carolina was nervous about this week. She felt that asking these questions on behalf of Kevin could help him and maybe other young people affected by the epidemic when people saw the film. She was also nervous about going to the prom with her boyfriend, a senior. We would finish our last interview with her, and she would immediately have to get her hair done and dress; there would be barely enough time.

We teased her about it then, but to her the prom was a big deal. So we promised to get her there on time.

The first of the three Carolina was to meet was Thoraya Obaid, the executive director of the United Nations Population Fund (UNFPA). I thought Ms. Obaid would be a very strong advocate for condom use, perhaps because I had met the company that did the condom testing for the UNFPA. I'd also seen her speak passionately on the issue of the prevalence of HIV/AIDS in women at the AIDS Conference in Bangkok.

We waited in the foyer, with an armed security guard. Carolina was in a denim jacket, slacks, and a T-shirt. Ms. Obaid came out in a tan business suit; she had curly short dark hair, and a wide face and smile. She was very friendly toward Carolina, who told her about her date and the prom. Ms. Obaid asked her if she had chosen her dress already. Carolina told her she had, and Ms. Obaid pressed, smiling, for more details. "Is it a long dress? Open?"

In the executive director's office, we finally sat down for Carolina's interview. Ms. Obaid told her about the increasing "feminization" of HIV/AIDS, how bad it was for young people, and particularly women. She had some literature for Carolina, and she showed her projects by young people about how to avoid AIDS. Carolina asked, "How can Kevin stay alive?"

"There is a formula to protect oneself and we call it the ABC. A for 'Abstinence' as long as you can, B for 'Be faithful,' meaning one partner, and C, 'Condom use.' This is the only way one can protect themselves from HIV/AIDS. And certainly this is the only approach that Kevin can do to protect himself."

Carolina asked her this question a few different ways, and abstinence was always put forth first by Ms. Obaid.

In the car, as we left, Carolina agreed with Sennye that she personally didn't think much of ABC. Even though it was what she was also being taught at school. But Carolina, like Kevin, was seventeen. She had bought a sexy dress for the prom, an annual event of young people with raging hormones.

And consider again this statistic from the UNFPA 2005 report: "Young people under the age of twenty-five represent almost a quarter of all people living with HIV. Half of all new HIV cases are among young people aged fifteen to twenty-four—with six thousand infected every day."

The next person we were to meet was Mary Robinson. She

had now started an independent NGO called Realizing Rights: The Ethical Globalization Initiative (EGI) to address, as their literature says, "three urgent issues required for greater human development and security: fostering more equitable international trade and development; strengthening responses to HIV/AIDS in Africa; and shaping more humane migration policies."

EGI's supporters included former U.S. president Jimmy Carter and Archbishop Desmond Tutu.

Carolina showed up in her denim jacket, writing her questions in the waiting room as we waited and read some of the speeches and papers Mary Robinson had written over the last few years.

Finally we were shown in.

Mary, a tall, striking woman, and, as she said, now a grandmother, told Carolina very sweetly that she was always happy to answer anything Kevin had to ask. She remembered his earlier questions from the AIDS Conference.

Carolina asked about abstinence versus condoms. Mary spoke about it from a human rights perspective, and came down much harder in favor of access to condoms than Thoraya Obaid had. She told Carolina that even when she was a lawyer in Ireland she had campaigned to let women have reproductive rights over their own bodies. Access to health care was a human right. As condoms were preventative measures to protect one's health, they were a right. She didn't think ABC was enough of a prevention measure. She related a story of a young Ethiopian woman she'd met who'd asked, "What about DEF?"

Carolina asked Mary what Kevin's rights were. She told Carolina about the Convention on the Rights of the Child. There were millions of children (like the ones we'd seen on the streets) living in abject poverty, without food, without health care, without education. However, with the exception of two countries—Somalia and the United States—all had signed this convention stating the rights of children, which were in line with the UN Declaration on Human Rights and the Child Rights Act of Kenya as well.

But?

But the world was not upholding those rights.

Carolina asked, on behalf of Kevin, what he could do. What was it that Kevin himself could do to protect his rights?

Mary said, "If there are others with him, they should form a little group. It's always better if you can be in a group. And he should know that if he can get his voice across, that human rights is on his side, the law is on his side, in fact, though he may not see that. And he should look for allies."

In other words, Kevin needed to organize himself.

He had rights. But unless he spoke up, got together with others, and/or reached out for allies, his rights would keep on being wronged.

I knew this answer on its own would just disappoint Kevin, so I asked Mary to do something special for him at the end of the interview.

Before I'd left Kisumu this last time, Kevin and I had gone into an Internet café. I'd left him with money (for everything) but also so that he could have access to e-mail, and I had asked the kind African lady at the counter, and the Indian couple who owned the café, if they could help Kevin set up an e-mail address. This way I could stay in touch with him, and he could write to other people.

Kevin had never touched a computer before. His first steps at it were very tentative. But he got himself an e-mail address at least.

On her little BlackBerry portable, as we stood there, Mary e-mailed the boy. She congratulated him on his hard work and told him she would be happy to let him know more about his rights.

The last person that Carolina would meet to ask Kevin's questions was Jeffrey Sachs. He was the author of *The End of Poverty,* a book with a foreword by Bono, calling Sachs his professor. Sachs was a key adviser to UN Secretary General Kofi Annan and was instrumental in overseeing the Millennium Development Goals, trying to eradicate extreme poverty—such as those Nairobi street children sniffing glue were experiencing—by the year 2025.

It was Friday afternoon, and Carolina was very nervous about missing her hair appointment. She wanted to look beautiful for her boyfriend at the prom.

We arrived at Columbia University and were met by Mary Tobin, Sachs's associate and press officer. He was busy at that moment, and, as we waited on the steps of the massive Grecian Low Library overlooking the campus, Carolina grew more and more nervous the longer he took to arrive. It was odd sitting here on the campus. This was my alma mater. I didn't feel much older than I had back then, and certainly not much wiser. And I was here with someone who was going to a prom. Funny old world.

Finally, Sachs arrived, in a plain dark suit. I appreciated the fact that he wasn't clean-shaven, but scruffy (as I often was). He and Carolina sat down on a stone wall overlooking the old campus. She told him they had to hurry. We had told her to tell Jeffrey Sachs why, so she explained that she had to get to the school prom. She said, "I know ending world poverty is important, but I want to go to the prom, too."

Sachs laughed. He scratched his chin. He acknowledged that was a tough one. Both were crucially important. So he said they would talk fast. She could fire away with the questions.

First, she asked one of her own. Remembering Mary Robinson's suggestion that he had to organize allies, she asked if Kevin was basically alone.

Sachs said something not unlike what Sujima, Senator Mechai's daughter, had said at the AIDS Conference. "Kevin is not alone because you care, I care, and I know millions of other people care. But Kevin can't depend on that alone. First he has to help himself, which he's doing, you know . . . he's fighting at school, he's fighting for survival, fighting for his future. And he's going to have to work together with his community. But we have to do more also. We have within our reach right now all these great breakthroughs to help Kevin, to help the communities where the Kevins all over Africa are living and struggling right now. Those communities can break out of poverty; they can get ahead but they need our help to do it and our governments need to follow through."

He talked about how much our governments promised, and how seldom they came through on their promises. Unfair agricultural subsidies. Aid that came through too late or too little. U.S. aid that benefited American companies, while at the same time creating debt for the recipients.

He told Carolina that this was her generation's homework assignment: to end poverty. Over the next twenty years they could do it. *And* it was an open-book assignment.

He was a passionate man, obviously wanting to make a difference.

Afterward, we drove back with Carolina and her father. She was very happy with how the interview had gone. But she was very late for her appointment. We drove straight to the hair salon, where her mother was waiting.

Carolina got her hair done.

She bought earrings.

She drove home.

She put on her makeup, and put on her white dress.

She went to the prom, and then away for the weekend with all her friends. And her boyfriend.

I did not ask her later what part of ABC, or DEF, they practiced.

CHAPTER FORTY

WHAT KEVIN LEARNED
FROM NEW YORK

On my return to Kenya after my trip to New York, I went with Kevin (on his last filming visit to Nairobi) to an Internet café. I could use the cheap "Internet" phone to call my lovely Sarah without feeling guilty about spending ninety-eight shillings a minute calling Australia (where she was now), maintaining contact with this patient woman I loved so many thousands of miles away.

Kevin sat with the proprietor of the shop to look at his e-mail. I came back while they were busy sorting it. Kevin was very happy to see the e-mail from Mary Robinson in his Inbox, and he e-mailed her back.

(Incidentally, she e-mailed back, too.)

Later, at Cathy's house, I showed Kevin the copy of the Convention on the Rights of the Child, which Pierre had printed out. There are fifty-four articles in it, covering liberty, health, nationalities—a wide spectrum of his rights. Kevin listened to what Mary Robinson had to say. He heard what Jeffrey Sachs had to say. He heard what Thoraya Obaid had to say. He knew they were very important, powerful people. He was grateful they had answered his questions.

The one thing he seemed to glean from these interviews was that, unless he organized himself, not much would happen. He took this information on board, and continued to mull it over, as he met three more people who would change his life and tell him more about what it was he had to do.

CHAPTER FORTY-ONE

A HAPPY ENDING FOR A STREET CHILD

One of the people Kevin met was a former street child, now a reformed young man. Anthony Lundi had taken Kevin to meet the director of the National Youth Service, in his military uniform complete with badges, and then to see what this "Youth Service" was all about. The NYS had been started shortly after the war for independence from the British. (Independence came in 1963.) Something had to be done for all the troops, all the young Kenyan fighters, who now needed something to keep them occupied. The NYS was created to give them military discipline and also a trade, such as auto mechanics, welding, and the like. Over the years, it had actually become quite prestigious, and now well-to-do families also wanted their young men and women to get into the program.

The vice president, working together with an industrialist with an interest in street children, Dr. Manu Chandaria, and other parties, had decided to try to rehabilitate some of the street children. Why not get some of them involved with the NYS? The program mixed them in with the other young people, not identifying who was a street youth and who not, so that they would not be discriminated against. As with all things, of course, there was criticism—some of it coming from the well-to-do families who now had fewer places for their own children.

But now Kevin and I watched these young people learning welding and how to fix cars. We watched them marching in the yard, as the late afternoon sun shone through the dust they kicked up.

We met three young men, all in uniform. All had formerly lived on the street. One was particularly lively, his eyes flashing as he spoke to Kevin. "Those days in the street, I was a bad man. I ganged up with other people to steal. And they wouldn't care if they killed someone." He said how some of his friends were arrested by the police and disappeared. He heard they'd gone into the National Youth Service. At first he'd thought that his friends were suffering badly, but then he'd heard that they were actually enjoying themselves, that they were getting fed and trained. So when he had a chance to get in himself, he'd jumped at it. He bathed. He wore clothes. He ate. He was learning a trade. "I've really changed now, you know. I don't even smoke."

Kevin asked him if when he was on the street he'd protected himself against AIDS. The young man told him he was so high on drugs, he hadn't even thought of that at the time. The street kids all figured they'd die anyway, so why put on a condom? Why protect yourself? Now, however, he would. He would.

He would not have been much older than Kevin, who was intimidated, and impressed.

I could imagine the young former street boy at that "river," sniffing glue, growing violent and tough with nothing to lose. Yet now here he was, polite and self-respecting. I'm not a military man by any means, but I was impressed. At that moment, whatever criticism anyone might have, I was witness to a human being who was now recognized as such, one who actually recognized himself as a human being. Here was a life actually changed. It gave us a sense of hope: change was possible.

There's a Jewish saying that if you save a life, you save a universe. With this young man, someone had saved a universe. It felt good to see.

CHAPTER FORTY-TWO
THE OTHER SIDE OF THE WORLD

There is another Nairobi, a Nairobi a world away from the squalor of the "river" or the worn-down '60s and '70s downtown center. This is a Nairobi of big, expensive houses, with fences and gates and guards, and grounds that go to the river—a very different river from that of the street children, a river that actually flows.

That was where we went next, courtesy of Lucy Yinda. Through her and Anthony Lundi, we were to meet Dr. Manu Chandaria, OBE, EBS. I knew little about him other than that he was a very rich and powerful industrialist in Kenya. He was so well known that even Kevin had heard his name. And, while Kevin didn't appear too nervous, he did know that a man like this could make a difference in his life. Somehow.

Within days of meeting the young man from the NYS, we drove with Cathy past embassies and large houses until we reached an impressive driveway leading to an impressive gate. We buzzed. We were let in. We drove through the grounds; beautiful lush tropical plants surrounding a lovely small meadow with waist-high stone walls, above which was a tasteful but modern house. There was a rustling in the trees—monkeys playing around. As Kevin waited, wandering around the grounds, I went to the house to let Dr. Chandaria's staff know we'd arrived.

A few minutes later, a short elderly Indian man in a gray sweater vest over a button-down shirt came buoyantly out of the house. He was probably in his seventies but his hair was still black, and he had such a twinkle in his eye that it was difficult to tell how old he really was. He greeted Kevin effusively. They stood and talked, a bit formally, a bit stiff at first. Dr. Chandaria asked about Kevin's ambitions, and the boy told him he wanted to go to university and become a doctor. Chandaria nodded. "That's fine, that's fine." He said he was on the board of Nairobi University. Kevin smiled. Chandaria smiled, too, putting a paternal hand on Kevin's shoulder. "If you get the good grades, then we'll get you in. So that you can be a doctor. But you have to have good grades. Are your grades good?"

Kevin, a bit embarrassed, told him how he had been fourth in his class, but that his grades had started slipping.

They came down to sit on the stone wall in the large garden below the house, and Chandaria told Kevin a bit about himself. How he had come from a poor family himself. (The English had brought Indians into Kenya as laborers at the beginning of the twentieth century, to build the railway line.) His mother and father had been illiterate, but Chandaria had done well at school. He had gone to America to study engineering at university. He had made something of himself. Now he was a well-known industrialist. He was on the board of many organizations, helping street children (as Kevin now knew), and talking to the government. Then Kevin told his story, and something appeared to shift for Dr. Chandaria. Seeming to trust the man, Kevin told him how he had been orphaned. How he lived alone.

"Who cooks for you?" the industrialist asked.

"I do," Kevin told him.

"And you wash your clothes?"

"Yes."

"And you go to school?"

"Yes."

Chandaria looked at me, somewhat shocked. "This is one of the special cases," he said.

"Does anybody at your school know about you? What you're going through?"

"No. I just . . . feel ashamed going as if you're advertising yourself to people, that 'I'm poor, I'm poor, I'm poor,'" Kevin replied.

Chandaria almost interrupted. "No, no, no. Poverty is not a crime. But if you don't talk, how can you find solutions? How would I know that you're poor?"

Chandaria told Kevin there were many rich people who could help, who should help. There was money in the governments. But they needed to know what was going on. They needed Kevin to tell them. "We need a voice of yours," he said.

Kevin seemed a bit stunned. Here he was talking with an enormously rich man, an enormously powerful man, who was saying that it was actually he who needed Kevin. Not the other way around. He asked Kevin if he knew whether there were other children orphaned at his school. Other children poor like him.

Kevin said there were. Most had relatives to help but still were poor.

Chandaria asked if he knew how many.

Kevin said he had not found out.

"Find out. Please find out. We want you to say what is going on. Why are you suffering? Do you think you should suffer?"

"No."

"So are you going to speak about it?"

Kevin nodded.

"We want a voice of yours. Are you going to get other orphans like you together? And make a loud noise?"

Kevin considered what Dr. Chandaria was saying.

The man's wife, a very petite Indian woman in a long blue gown, came to watch. Her husband was extremely animated. He was telling Kevin they needed to hear what it was like for children like him to suffer. There were hundreds of thousands of children in Kenya living on the streets. If they could find out the orphans who were really needy at Kevin's school, his organization could do something for the children. His school could be a test case.

Finally, Kevin looked at him seriously and said, "I'll do it. I'll do it."

"Are you sure? Sure, Kevin?"

Kevin nodded.

They shook hands on it.

We went inside the house for tea and biscuits. Chandaria took Kevin upstairs to show him his office. Kevin told Chandaria about whom he was meeting next; a man he was very nervous to meet. Chandaria went into his bedroom. Kevin followed. The industrialist went into his closet, where there were only about five suits (for a man as wealthy as he was, this came as a surprise). He took out one beautiful dark suit and handed it to Kevin, saying, "As a memory from me, you can take this with you, so that you can wear a nice suit."

He looked at Kevin, motioning from his head to Kevin's head, a full head higher. "We're almost the same height. The same height more or less. Now wear nicely and look good . . . and smart, huh?"

Kevin came downstairs with his new suit, happy beyond belief.

Downstairs, we talked for a while with his wife, in front of a painting of Mother Teresa, a painting that had been autographed for Chandaria by Mother Teresa herself. She was someone he'd come to know quite well. He told us about meeting Jeffrey Sachs and telling him how the corruption in Kenya had to stop, that business leaders in Africa had to get involved in their communities.

I think at that moment all Kevin could see was his new suit.

CHAPTER FORTY-THREE
KEVIN WEARS THE SUIT

There was a reason that Kevin would need a suit. He had been wearing his red flannel shirt most days, partly because it was one of the few pieces of clothing he owned but also because for him Nairobi was still chilly. But he had a meeting the next afternoon with someone he wanted to look especially smart for, someone whom he very much wanted to impress and felt honored to be meeting: the vice president of Kenya, the man directly in charge of all of the orphans in Kenya.

(We could have met with the first lady, but she was in political hot water for getting into a major squabble with the press. And the new president of Kenya was at the center of too much corruption talk as well. The one person everyone could say no wrong about then was the vice president. And that's whom Kevin was to meet.)

The suit.

Kevin tried on the jacket in his room at Cathy's in front of the two of us. It literally fitted perfectly. Then he asked us to leave for a bit of privacy, so he could try on the pants. We waited outside, and then came back in when he called us. The trousers were perhaps made for Chandaria at a time when he was much plumper than he was now. We could have had them tailored but not in time for the meeting with the vice president.

Cathy's husband, Jim, let Kevin try on a pair of his pants, as well as a nice white shirt.

They fitted. The tie was from Chandaria.

Again, Cathy and I withdrew, but then were called in by the extraordinarily proud and grinning Young Man Wearing a Dark Blue Suit. It would do. It would do very well.

CHAPTER FORTY-FOUR

KEVIN MEETS THE VICE PRESIDENT

And so that afternoon, Young Man Wearing a Dark Blue Suit walked out of Longonot Place toward the Norfolk Hotel, where the beautiful old English-style taxis waited. A taxi driver held the door open for Young Man Wearing a Dark Blue Suit, who climbed into the back, followed by his team.

And off we went.

In the taxi was a sign: "With God, all things are possible."

Kevin was something far beyond nervous, staring straight ahead.

I told him it would be fine.

He nodded. He didn't believe me.

I told him he should believe me. After all, hadn't everything worked out fine to date with every person he'd met?

He still didn't believe me.

To lighten his nerves, I told him a story I'd read long ago about an African leader in a small country who was so taken with himself that he awarded himself a massive number of honorary titles: His Most Eminent Graceful and Sublime, the Great and Distinguished Most Benevolent Vastness, Emperor of All That Is And Ever Was, Ruler Sanctimonious Beyond . . .

Kevin giggled.

I asked Kevin, just so, to refer to me henceforth as Most Excellent Excellency. He said, "Of course, Your Most Excellent Excellency. And Cathy?"

Cathy wanted to be called "Her Ladyship."

Kevin liked that. But I still don't know if he believed me that it would be all right.

We had still to settle on an honorific for him when we arrived at Jogoo House on Harambee Avenue, where the vice president's office was located.

Kevin got out of the taxi. The driver said he would wait for us. We told the guards outside we were there to see the vice president. Kevin was very serious; Cathy and I were smiling. We were let through.

We climbed various flights of dark stairs, asking for directions as we went. Young Man Wearing a Dark Blue Suit walked up to the gated window, where two guards in dark blue official uniform were standing, one younger than the other.

Kevin said, "Hello. I'd like to speak to the vice president."

The younger guard asked if he had an appointment.

Kevin nodded.

Eventually he was let through. The older guard smartly saluted Kevin as he passed.

We were shown into a waiting area, where there was another

camera crew waiting. I assumed they must be there to film the vice president as well, either before or after us.

Cathy was greeted by Browne Kutswa, his press representative, the man with whom she'd been working so hard to set up this interview. He shook hands with Kevin, then me, and said it would just be a little while.

Kevin was nervous. I was nervous—for Kevin and for the film. Kevin wasn't a hardened journalist. He was a kid with no one to really back him up in this country. Even his old counselor, Joseph, now worked for another AIDS agency, and Kevin hadn't seen him in a while. Politicians are renowned for making all the right noises but not necessarily following through on their words. Would the vice president disappoint Kevin?

The other camera crew looked over our camera admiringly. They had a nice, bigger but older camera.

Eventually Browne Kutswa came and told us we were ready to go. We said good-bye to the other camera crew and started off down the hall, filming Kevin as he made his big entrance into the office. We walked down the hall and pushed through into the office of the Honorable A. Moody Awori. Then, with Browne Kutswa showing the way, Kevin went ahead to greet the vice president. We followed him through the reception area, past the two women sitting at their desks, into a larger office.

At the back of that wood-and-leather-paneled office sat an older man with a round face and crinkly eyes, and wearing a light blue shirt and tie. He stood up at his desk and extended his hand. "Kevin, is it?"

Kevin came over with a huge smile, took his hand, and just kept shaking it.

And kept shaking it.

They sat at the desk, and the vice president asked him how he was. Kevin told him he was fine. Dr. Awori had a mellifluous voice and a slow but charming smile. He asked Kevin to tell him about his life. He listened to his story intently, asking questions, praising him for wanting to become a doctor.

At that point the other camera crew came in and began to set up on the opposite side of the room, where we were going to do our interview and where Cathy and I were busy setting up. I was about to protest that we hadn't yet done our filming. It turned out that they were there to film us filming the vice president and Kevin!

That was quite convenient. They lit the scene for us and helped us get our shot together as well.

It was time for the interview to begin, and Kevin and Dr. Moody Awori sat in their appointed seats opposite each other.

Kevin told him that he had been interviewing world leaders—meaning of course that his questions had been asked of world leaders—and asked, "As a leader, how has the AIDS epidemic affected you?"

Dr. Awori told Kevin that, for the last twenty-five years, AIDS had been killing about seven hundred people a day in Kenya. "The whole way of life is changed completely." As a leader, he wanted to have his people healthy. He wanted to see people living well. He didn't want to see children orphaned. "As a leader I do not want to see children without their parents. Right now there are estimated to be 1.5 million orphans in Kenya."

And then our roving journalist asked, straight on, "Concerning 1.5 million orphans in Kenya, what plan does the government have to make sure they are well taken care of?"

Dr. Awori replied, "We, as Africans, must find an African solution. It's no longer tenable for us to expect that people will come from somewhere to come and assist us. So the first thing to know is that we are on our own."

He talked to Kevin about some of the programs the young man had already heard of and seen, such as the National Youth Service, about primary schools, about the bursary fund (that the MPs were stealing from). The vice president talked about nutrition and how people needed to eat better. If they were healthier, that would help to combat the AIDS epidemic. He spoke about how Kenya needed to get rid of poverty.

Dr. Awori also told Kevin that they needed to find a return to family values.

My heart sank, having heard that phrase so often in America, where to me it often seemed to mean cutting back monies allocated to social welfare. But he then qualified his words, emphasizing that he meant African family values. He was very clear on that. For thousands of years, people in Africa had survived before colonization and Western medicine. Communities had taken care of each other.

He talked about an idea in its formative stages, in which he surmised that, out of a population of, say, thirty million people, there were around eight to ten million families. With

1.5 million orphans, if each family would take one, and the government contributed to their care, that could alleviate or solve the crisis of the AIDS epidemic. He did not talk about abstinence or condoms.

But then, just as Chandaria and Robinson had done, he put the focus back on Kevin. "And you as a person, what do you think is your role, apart from interviewing world leaders and so forth . . . what is the action that you think you can take and others like yourself to help?"

What could Kevin do?

Kevin just stared at him. Yet one more person asking him what he was going to do about the epidemic and orphans.

We eventually said our good-byes. I'm not sure at this point that Kevin actually thought about what the vice president had said. He was just starry-eyed from having met him.

Browne Kutswa told us that apparently we would be on the next day's news. On KBC, Kenyan Broadcasting Corporation.

Kevin, the orphan from Kisumu, who'd lived alone in a shack for so many years, would now be seen on national television asking the vice president what he was doing about the AIDS epidemic and orphans.

The older guard saluted Kevin as we were graciously allowed to leave the building.

"Thank you," Kevin said.

That day this nutritionist okayed chicken and French fries for dinner! And Kevin was pleased, very pleased, with the vice president—and himself.

I learned later from people who'd been at government meetings over the next few days that the vice president referred often to his meeting with Kevin, impressed at having met such a remarkable young man, from such difficult circumstances.

CHAPTER FORTY-FIVE

ORPHANS REUNITED WITH SEVENTH DAY ADVENTIST CHICKEN

Before we left Nairobi for good on this film, Kevin, Cathy, and I drove to the Seventh Day Adventist school to rescue Ann and Evelyn, as promised, from "the scourge" of vegetarian food and indulge in congratulatory chicken and French fries at the Village Market nearby. As we drove, they wanted to know excitedly how Kevin had fared with the vice president. And he told them all about it, proudly, but still shy amidst their female company.

In the posh, swanky food courts, Ann and Evelyn, followed by Kevin, took a quick look and bypassed all the various German, Thai, and Italian establishments and went straight to the stall with the big "Grilled Meats" sign. I went off to find a present for Kevin's teacher, Joy, who had been so kind in helping us coordinate his schedule and in watching out for him as well. I couldn't have been gone very long, but by the time I returned,

Ann and Evelyn were engrossed in their chicken and French fries (yes, and Coke; "Always Coca Cola" in Kenya—literally). They were ravenous.

They spoke a little differently to Kevin now. Not because of his "access" to the vice president and "world leaders," but because he himself was different, not as painfully shy anymore. There was a bit more play and confidence in his demeanor. He didn't rush through his food, more interested in chatting with the two of them whenever they came up for air. Finally, as they drew closer to finishing their meal, Ann and Evelyn transformed back into the demure girls Kevin had initially met. They, too, had changed over the years since I'd met them; they had poise, self-assurance. Ann no longer just wanted to be a nurse. No longer just a doctor either, as Kevin did. Now she wanted to be a surgeon!

As I watched these three young people I'd come to care about far more than I'd first bargained for (before Sarah's original "voice in my ear")—and felt touched that the two girls told Kevin they called me "father"—I saw again what a role the love Ann and Evelyn had received from Lucy Yinda had played in their lives. Looking at them, I couldn't believe that these were two former street girls, one having to ply herself sexually for money, the other addicted to drugs. Lucy (truly their mother now) had given them a gift far superior to that of school fees. It was a gift she was giving to so many children at her Wema Centre: she loved them unconditionally. And each and every one of them felt that love individually, even if, like all teens, they may at times have wanted to rebel. They knew she loved them.

And that made them believe that, to paraphrase my nephew, "the ocean had arms." And those arms could hold them.

Later than we should have, with darkness settling on the road, we drove Ann and Evelyn back to their school. They gave Kevin big farewells—obvious affection shared amongst all of them. I remembered the conversation when Kevin and Ann had first met and sat on the grassy field. She'd said, "Do you intend to be alone for the rest of your life?"

"No, I'm planning to get married and have a family."

"Well," she'd said, hmmphing, "do you want to marry an orphan just like you so that she can understand your problems, or do you want to get a girl who comes from high places, like a rich girl?"

He had been embarrassed. "That one I can't tell because, you know, love is blind. You may get attracted to an orphan, yeah? So I can't tell now." And he'd given a bashful smile.

There was another one now as the girls walked away into the night.

CHAPTER FORTY-SIX
KEVIN LEAVES THE BIG CITY

It was Kevin's last night in Nairobi. Jim and Cathy had to go out to a function for Jim's work. I had thought I would take Kevin out to a nightclub. He could listen to music and discover dancing. And he could just have fun! He was about to go back to school after all.

However, that was not to be. Not this night.

We had little time left before we came to the end of filming. Kevin knew my visits would soon become infrequent, as I would be based once again in Australia or elsewhere, unable to afford these frequent trips to Kisumu. So he was not so interested in exploring the outside world this evening. That he could do in the future. Right now, there were two more interviews that had to be done. One was by me of him. That was to be the easy and simple one. The other one would be Kevin's interview of me.

The aim of the first one was this: I wanted to see if everything we'd gone through in the past months—discussions of abstinence, condoms, abstinence, condoms . . . ad nauseam—had changed Kevin's point of view at all.

I said, "Kevin, we've been doing this for a long time now. And we've talked to a lot of people, in Kenya, Thailand, Australia, the United States, and even Swizzerland [which was how he pronounced Switzerland]."

He smiled.

I continued. "At first, people said to you, 'Don't use condoms, God will be very angry.' So now, what has Kevin learned?"

Kevin thought a moment and then said, "Okay. If it is a must that you have sex, then you have to put on the . . . [he paused] . . . is it the *fucking* condom?"

I burst into paroxysms of laughter. As did he. He had never cursed or used that word before in all the time I'd known him (though I had!). But in this context, he was right. "Yes," I said, "it's the fucking condom."

"If I can say it so," he giggled. "But my principle is to abstain until I get married."

"But if you don't?"

He was very serious. "No, I won't have sex."

"Kevin, I don't believe you."

"Believe me. Believe me!"

This went on and on until, finally, I said quietly, "Will you promise me, Kevin, if you do have sex before you get married, what will happen?"

He took a moment. "Okay. If emotion drives me crazy, then I'll have to . . . I . . . I will put on the fucking condom."

"Amen," I said.

"And you, too, Miles."

We burst into laughter again. I was proud of him.

At this point, we were still going to go out and get dinner, and then move on to the nightclub. I only had one more thing I needed Kevin to do. I had arranged through the various financing sources for him to receive a substantial amount of money by Kenyan standards. But those sources of course wanted him to sign a piece of paper saying he had received it. I knew we would have to write it together, so I explained this to him.

He looked at me, immediately withdrawing into some place of pain that I didn't understand. "But you look out for me, Miles."

"Of course," I replied. But, I told him, I wanted him to be taken care of, if something did happen to me. "Just in case," I said. I couldn't give him all the money to keep in his shack. He'd already been robbed—just of schoolbooks. (He agreed with that.) He was too young and didn't have the right papers to open a bank account. And I feared that, because of his tender nature, he could easily be swindled by someone. (He agreed with that, too.) We couldn't give the money to the people in his community, as they were needy themselves. (He also agreed with that.) So the idea was to give it to Frederik and Nathalie from Kisumu, who'd watched out for him all these years and who had plenty of their own resources. They would hold it for him. And he and I were just writing this agreement so that, in case something happened to me, he had proof this was his money. Nathalie and Frederik would sign it, too.

"But what would happen to you?"

"I don't know," I said, "but *if*—"

He burst into tears, tears of abandonment, tears of reproach, tears of sorrow I had never seen from him before.

"You are abandoning me," he cried.

Over and over he said that I was abandoning him.

I realized finally what he meant. His father had died of HIV/AIDS. He had "abandoned" him. His mother had died three years later. She had "abandoned" him. Now I was hinting that I might do the same. Even though I would be leaving him a substantial amount of money, so he wouldn't have to worry, and which would see him through his schooling. And even though I reminded him how Dr. Chandaria had promised to pay for his university, to get him an interview with the board. And even though he had met so many influential people who would promise to help him, because they knew of his plight now.

"You want to abandon me. After all this time," he said to me. (Cathy had said to me that for Kevin there was life pre-Miles, and life post-Miles. And one was better.) Weeping, he told me I had been like his mother and father, since he didn't have them—even though I was so far away.

I came over to him and tried to hold him as I could only imagine his mother or father might have. I tried to be the ocean's arms.

I promised I would not abandon him.

When he had settled down, he told me that, like Ann and Evelyn, he wanted to go to boarding school. He knew I could not stay in Kenya, but he did not want to live alone anymore.

And I apologized to him. I told him I could have made his life so much better in these last years. It wasn't just that I hadn't been told. He had seemed so attached to his mother's blue and brown chairs that I had felt he could not leave them. I had asked him once when he had been very much younger why he didn't sell them. He had looked at me point-blank and said, "They're my mother's."

Kevin had said he wanted to stay on his own. (But I should have known better, despite what his various community leaders might have said.)

He kindly replied, "You didn't know. They didn't tell you."

Then, in all seriousness, he quietly said, "But I would like to go to boarding school now. I don't want to be alone."

I said again I would not abandon him. (Neither would Cathy, Joy, Lucy Yinda, Frederik and Nathalie, and all the other people committed to him, like little Julia in Swizzerland. We would try to show that the universe did have arms.)

He said, "Thank you, Your Most Excellent Excellency."

And I realized what his honorific would be, this boy who had impressed me, and so many others, with even the vice president referring to him in his meetings. His honorific should be: Mr. President.

"No, thank *you*, Mr. President."

CHAPTER FORTY-SEVEN

SOME HAPPY ENDINGS

We flew back to Kisumu to enjoy a few more days together. Kevin was going to return to the people he'd met at the beginning of our journey to see what had happened to them. Then, he was going to go to his school where he would try to heed the advice of Mary Robinson and Dr. Chandaria—even of Dr. Awori, the vice president.

We went back to his shack, which he was planning to leave soon. We saw Albert, his neighbor, there and talked to him. Kevin was in his smart red school suit. Albert wore a white T-shirt and a FedEx cap. In the small slum in Kisumu, Kevin told him that he had met many people since they had first spoken. He had talked to them about abstinence and condoms.

Albert nodded, nicely. And in the small slum in Kisumu, Kevin said, "Recently I even spoke to the vice president of Kenya."

Albert nodded and said, "Uh-huh."

Kevin continued, "Many people are saying the best way to protect yourself is with a condom."

Albert explained to him about the will of God.

He also said he should stop thinking so much about condoms and instead needed to study in school.

I saw how well-meaning Albert was toward Kevin, how he wanted him to do well. The little he knew was the myth he had been told: not to wear condoms but to pray. Kevin seemed to see this now, too.

I did not get to see Edwina again on this trip, but I was told she was doing well and still lecturing pregnant mothers. We left her some money through Kevin. And it gave her some relief, he later told me. She'd been very happy about that. (We have stayed in touch since then, and, brave young woman that she is, she is now taking care of the same mother that she'd said would not take care of her.)

Kevin, now very concerned about others, went back to see Jane's children. He wanted to see how they were holding up, as the father would most probably still be alive.

We walked through the mud, past stray chickens and a few thin cows to a familiar clay shack with a corrugated roof. When we knocked on the shack door, there was a shuffling of feet. Kevin called out, "Hello."

A woman's voice asked him to hold on.

"It's Kevin," he added.

The sound of shuffling feet grew closer. Out of the darkness of the shack emerged a tall, strong woman in an orange dress.

"Jane?" Kevin asked.

I didn't recognize her, either. I had been sure she was going to die. To "abandon" her children to "God."

It was Jane. She had some small growths on her skin and a bump on her chin, but she was very very much alive.

She and Kevin sat down; he smiled profusely. He said later, "I couldn't believe how Jane looked. I told her how happy I was to see her. She told me she had been taking ARVs. But I couldn't believe this was Jane."

To show him how healthy she was, she jumped up from her chair and even danced a few steps and sang. She said, "I have energy. See, I can walk. I can jump."

Mr. President was so happy, so happy. The medicine had worked.

The medicine *worked.*

Chapter Forty-eight
ORPHANS OF THE WORLD, UNITE!

A few months later, toward the end of 2005, I woke up in a worried mood, which turned to foul as the day went on. It was raining outside, a rarity in Australia, and the wind was beating down outside our apartment close to the famous Bondi Beach.

I was having what parents of teenagers refer to as "a melt-down." My darling Sarah tried to be sympathetic, and tell me everything would work out. But I felt that nothing I'd been working on over these past few years would bear fruit. I felt use-less: in the face of this epidemic, as a storyteller, as a human being. What value had my life? Nothing had changed. I could yammer on and on about the AIDS epidemic, get uninvited to any friends' dinners, and still not raise money for more efforts. What value had my life?

I went upstairs and played myself the videotape of the speech Kevin had made to the orphans at his school.

When we had returned to Kisumu that last time, Kevin had gone and spoken to the principal of the school. He told him that he had met Dr. Chandaria and thought that perhaps Chandaria could help some of the other orphans at the school. The principal was a bit disbelieving at first—as anyone might be. Dr. Chandaria is a legendary household name in Kenya. But he told Kevin that, out of a school of 1200 boys, 300 were orphans.

. There were many to help.

Kevin began to speak to small groups of these young men, to talk to them and see how they were feeling. In the courtyard, in classrooms, in hallways. He had things he wanted to say to them. It wasn't easy. Many orphans wouldn't, couldn't, come out and admit that they were indeed orphans. There were many who were not orphans who felt they needed help, too. In one classroom of schoolboys, a few gathered at the end of the day as it rained outside to talk about these issues. "Why should only orphans get help?" one asked. Another boy talked about how his father was taking care of many nieces and nephews. Although he was not an orphan, his family needed help in caring for all these children who were. Kevin said he thought the boy had a point. But at least, at the very least, he argued, this boy had parents who could try on his behalf.

One afternoon, in the school gymnasium, a whole group of young teenage men—boys in their red jackets and ties—gathered together a bunch of chairs so they could sit and listen to Kevin speak. He stood waiting as they gradually made less and less clatter with their chairs and settled down.

This was the young man who, when I had first met him, could barely speak; a boy in a shack through which a chicken wandered freely, a chicken that was far louder than the boy. This was a boy who could not stand to look at his mother's photographs, who could not admit that she had died of AIDS because of stigmatization.

And this is what he said—The President.

Good evening.

I'm Kevin. And I've been going around asking world leaders about the rights of orphans, and even I talked to them about AIDS. I have a few things that I've learned that I would like to share with you. And I hope at the end it can make a change in our lives.

First, we are all orphans, isn't it? And we as orphans, we undergo very difficult experiences. I'm sure if I start asking everyone's experience, if you told the experience, you will just find your tears rolling down. You find that at some places our rights are being abused, because we don't have our parents. But what I learned, as orphans, we have rights like any other children. And you have to know your rights.

And also I discussed with organizations' executive directors about AIDS and how to prevent it. You know, we are approaching our adolescent stage, and that sexual urge, sometimes it can drive you crazy. The way to prevent yourself is that you either abstain, or if you can't abstain, you have to use condoms. But you know condoms, it's not 100 percent sure. Sometimes you can use it and it ruptures and a whole mess comes into your life.

Stigmatization on AIDS is very rampant. If you have AIDS, you can't express it freely. For fear that you'll either be rejected in the community or people won't associate with you. People will begin saying maybe that one was a prostitute or something of that sort. So if someone has AIDS, even your neighbors, you don't need to have to fear your neighbor. You just have to be friendly to him or her, because AIDS is just like malaria or any other disease. You don't need to stigmatize such a person by insulting her. You just have to be friendly and accept him or her.

As an orphan, let's say your parents die of AIDS, and maybe you got infected through one way or the other, you should not just keep quiet. Because now there are some organizations wishing to help orphans who are infected by giving them medicine that can prolong their lives. So if you're infected, you don't have to keep quiet that I'm an orphan, I'll be laughed at. You have to express yourself out so that you can get help.

I met Dr. Manu Chandaria and talked a great deal with him. And Dr. Chandaria told me that when I come back to Kisumu, we have to mobilize ourselves as orphans. Such that we can get at least some help.

He gave me the example of when someone has a problem and he cries out, few people will hear him. Some will even ignore him and go their way. But when suppose around ten people have such a problem and they cry out, their voice will be louder. So by mobilizing orphans, let's say we write to the government. When the government sees a list of one hundred orphans, they will have to put a question mark why. When you're a good number, people and government will at least take consideration what is happening and they'll have to try and help.

As for me, I have gone under very difficult situations. And some of you here have gone under very difficult situations. So we have to join our hands to see that all our needs are met. So that we can work together and get help. So are you willing to join hands?

"Yes," said a few boys in the room. Quietly at first.

Kevin asked again.

"Yes," they all said in unison.

"Yes," I said, sitting thousands of miles away. I asked Sarah, sitting beside me.

"Yes," said Sarah, emphatically.

Epilogue

AND NOW

And Now......
Here is a recent email I received from Kevin.

Dear Miles,

Receive greetings from Mr. President and hopes that all is fine wherever you are.

I'm very happy to hear from you and much to hear that my fee [for boarding school] is already paid.

Thank once again for the storybooks. I really enjoyed them, and the dictionary for it has become handy.

Miles, I really miss you and Cathy, and I keep wondering when will we be together again?

Pass greetings to all and to Sarah with much love from Mr. President.

I really miss your company, too.

From Kevin,

With love.

Through the efforts of so many—Cathy; Kevin's teacher, Joy; Veronica; and Julia, of course—Kevin is now boarding at his school. (Who knew it would be so hard to get into the boarding program even with the money for his fees?) It was only for the last quarter of the school year, and the fee was the same as if for the whole year. But Kevin had nearly not even managed that. He had become badly ill with pneumonia. Luckily he had been recording voice-over for the film with Cathy, who got him medical care, and when she had to leave for Australia, he stayed a week in Nairobi with Lucy Yinda's sister.

But even so, back in Kisumu, Kevin e-mailed me and said that he thought the boarding fee for the quarter was too expensive (even though we'd be paying for it); perhaps it could help another orphan. I had e-mailed Mr. President and told him that if he got sick again on his own, who would speak for the orphans? It was time for him to be taken care of now.

He spent Christmas with Cathy and Jim in Nairobi, and they bought him swimming lessons. He started learning that water can have arms, and could hold him. He had roast chicken with vegetables.

Then he started the year at boarding school. Ironically, although he enjoyed the company, his grades suffered. And he asked if he could return home to get the grades he would need to become a doctor. To which, as he called me his mother and father, I assented.

He graduated with a B+ average. It's just under what the universities are requiring, but we have applied and Dr. Chandaria did write his letter as promised. For a boy who raised himself from the age of 10, it's not bad. I'm proud of him.

And through the kind graces of Sean Emery and the University of New South Wales, he was offered a trip to Australia to attend another AIDS conference. We got him a passport now that he was eighteen, and a visa. Australia is where he is right now. With Sarah for the first time. I am about to join them.

And I think about a walk I did along the beach there, where I saw a young whale breach . . .

Our film together was well received. One review said: "As many people as possible should watch it, strapped down *A Clockwork Orange*-style if necessary. Great stuff." Another said: "Kevin's story makes the staggering global HIV/AIDS figures, and the heartbreak felt by the 15 million AIDS orphans, painfully real."

His story touched viewers, many of whom wrote in wanting to help. Some of their letters, in which they admitted how hard they cried, brought tears to my eyes. Kevin's story changed how they viewed this epidemic.

I am now working on a feature film about it. My hardworking feature-film producers and I speak every day, diligently trying to make our film about these children, children like Kevin.

I've said this to friends, and some don't believe me—but as Kevin said to me, "Believe me!"—that these brave children I've met, particularly Kevin, have changed me at least as much as I may have changed them. Kevin has changed me. I care far more than I ever thought I would about someone so many thousands of miles from where I live but, as I remember thinking about Father Michael, very close to home.

Life can be very difficult at times—for all of us. "Very lonely," as Kevin said. It can often *appear* that the ocean, the universe, does not have arms; that we will fall through the cracks. That feeling, which I remember well as a child, can be even stronger and meaner sometimes now that I'm an adult. But remembering that boy, my care for him and his for me, allows me to feel the universe's arms, if you will, and how far they can stretch.

Whether inspired by Buddha, Jesus, Moses, Mohammed, any divinity, our neighbors, or our own human spirit, we need to be the arms of the universe now and hold all these children at least until they can swim, and beyond if necessary. For their sake and ours. The AIDS epidemic has created the need for us to gather together in a way that I certainly have never heard of before, to reach out to these fifteen million stigmatized children. To reach out to the little street child in the box; to Humphrey, proudly surviving; to Pin in Thailand, singing her "Carrot Song." To reach out, as Kevin says in his email, "With Love."

Does it matter to anyone
if there is one less of us?

Does it matter if any
of us live or die?

Of course it does.
Just ask Kevin.

By buying this book you have already contributed to Kevin's education. For more information on how you can help children like Kevin, please visit:

www.makeitrealtome.com

ACKNOWLEDGMENTS

I would like to thank all those who have made this book possible. For their invaluable assistance in the making of these films (and the next one): Cathy Scott, her husband, Jim Terrie, Veronica Sive, Pierre Peyrot, Anna Laffy, Véronique Gauvin, David Jowsey, Sonya Pemberton, Cynthia Kane, Christian Vesper, Paola Freccero, Deirbhile ni Churraighin, Sumonpan Kosonsiriset, Julia Overton, Richard Brennan, Steven Corvini, the Australian Film Commission, Film Victoria, the Sundance Channel, TG4 (Ireland), Channel 11 Thailand, and the Australian Broadcasting Corporation, Christian Jacks, Beatrice Spadicini, James Cairns, Wanjuhi Kamau, Lara von Ahleveldt and Adam Wakeling of 3DD, Patty Buteux van der Kamp of Wanted Films, Anthony Lundi, Frederik and Nathalie Eijkman, Lucy Yinda, Xoliswa Sithole, Graham Bradstreet, Oliver Mtukudzi (for allowing us to use his music), Tony "Thunder" Smith, Keri Douglas, Marten

Rabarts, Charles Liburd, Joao Costa, Joy Akoyi (Kevin's teacher), Browne Kutsa, Catherine Vogel, Simon Prisk, Andrew Lambert, Chris Hennessey . . .

All those who have participated in the films: Carolina Réal, Ponlapat Charoonrasamichote, Julia Vogel, Sennye Mugale, Maxwell D. Nhlato, Mary Robinson, Jeffrey Sachs, Thoraya Obaid, Dennis Altman, Roger Short, Steve Wesselingh, David Cooper, Sean Emery, John Gerofi, Richard Muga, Charity Ngilu, David Awori, Manu Chandaria, Millie Odhiambo, A.B.C Ocholla, Father D'Agostino, Francis Otwane, Christopher Murray, David Reddy, Mechai Viravaidya, Arthorn Prachanat . . .

All those who have participated in the creation of this book: Gareth St John Thomas, Benny St. John Thomas, Anouska Jones, Christa Moffitt, Sadie Chrestman, Don Weise, John Sherer, Michele Jacob, Michael Walters, Michael Fedison, and Kay Mariea . . .

I'd also like to thank Archbishop Desmond Tutu for his extraordinarily kind support and his courage in his fight against injustice and the AIDS epidemic.

All who are courageously struggling and have struggled in their communities: Edwina Atieno, Joseph Musyoka, Jane Musyoka, Nixon Musyoka, Peter Ochola, Jane Ochola, and their children . . .

The extraordinary children (some of whom have grown up now!): Valentine Achiengi, Jimmy, Ann Njeri, Evelyn Shiro, Humphrey, Pin, Nixon, and every one of you.

My father, mother, brother, and sister, for watching over me.

Those of you whom I may have omitted to mention, I thank you for everything you've done for me and for these children. And forgive the omission. It's only an oversight as we rush to print.

I want to thank my love, Sarah Lambert, who has taught me that the universe does indeed have arms. No matter how far apart we may be, your voice is ever in my ear.

And most of all, extraordinary thanks to Kevin Sumba, a.k.a. Mr. President. Much love from a man attempting excellent Excellency.